PARASITES AND PARASITIC DISEASES

SCHISTOSOMIASIS

EPIDEMIOLOGY, DIAGNOSIS AND TREATMENT

PARASITES AND PARASITIC DISEASES

Additional books in this series can be found on Nova's website under the Series tab.

Additional e-books in this series can be found on Nova's website under the e-book tab.

PARASITES AND PARASITIC DISEASES

SCHISTOSOMIASIS

EPIDEMIOLOGY, DIAGNOSIS AND TREATMENT

ADRIANA ERICA MIELE
EDITOR

NOVA BIOMEDICAL

New York

For permission to use material from this book please contact us:
Telephone 631-231-7269; Fax 631-231-8175
Web Site: http://www.novapublishers.com

Library of Congress Cataloging-in-Publication Data

Library of Congress Control Number: 2014930033

ISBN: 978-1-63117-186-4

Published by Nova Science Publishers, Inc. † New York

Contents

Preface

Schistosomiasis, also known as bilharzia, is a very old parasitic disease, which has affected humans possibly all throughout their evolution. The oldest paleontological evidence comes from the fossilized eggs in ancient Egypt mummies. In their medical papyrus the "âaâ" disease, which results in red urines, is a gift of Seth to the Pharaohs. Similar descriptions have been found in tablets from Mesopotamia, of about the same period.

This long time of co-evolution has let the parasite, a multicellular organism belonging to the platyhelminth worms, to adapt to several different environments, and to become one of the least deadly of the human parasitic diseases, though one of the most disabling.

Schistosome parasite is a terrific example of successful hijacking of the human defense machinery: the worm enters through intact skin, undergoes two metamorphoses and reaches its final destination, in the veins either around the liver or around the bladder, completely undisturbed. The worm is able to switch off the innate immunity and to change the setup of the acquired immunity, switching it to a complete Th2 phenotype, as only auto-immune and allergic diseases are able to do.

The final destination is not chosen by chance: both the portal and vesical plexuses are among the richest veins in terms of nutrients (e.g., red blood cells and metabolites) and those with the slowest flux. Once attached to those veins, the blood-feeder adult worm couple (another peculiarity is that Schistosomes are not hermaphrodite worms, but digeneans) can live undisturbed for as long as thirty years.

Although the life cycle of Schistosome has been known for more than one hundred years, the disease is still affecting a huge part of the population living in tropical and sub-tropical area, and it is still endemic in 78 countries, where an estimated 243 million people required treatment. Schistosomiasis is second only to malaria per number of infected people, nevertheless it remains one of the most neglected among the tropical transmissible diseases.

Since the parasite requires an intermediate host snail living in warm freshwater, people get infected due to those activities linked to water, such as agriculture, fishing, recreational and domestic activities. Communities with poor access to drinking water and lacking sanitation are the most vulnerable, earning schistosomiasis the name of poverty-related disease. In particular, women and children are among the most affected patients. Moreover migration to urban areas and refugee movements are changing the geographical distribution of the disease.

In recent times, travelers and migrants are increasing the number of symptomatic cases in the northern hemisphere. They are not always promptly diagnosed, due both to inexperience of the health professionals and to clinical signs common to other helminthic diseases.

The World Health Organization has recently launched a mass drug administration program, which has lead to administer the drug of choice, praziquantel, to about 28.1 million people in 2011, selected among school-aged children and entire communities living in highly endemic areas. Despite this is an impressive number, it only represents one tenth of the infected population. Therefore the WHO has called for help from partners in order to find adequate funding to cure 100 million children world-wide. This is a huge call also on terms of manufacturing the praziquantel tablets, but it is necessary since most of the chronic effects of schistosomiasis leave irreversible signs in those patients, including stunted growth and impairment of cognitive function.

In recent times strong commitments have been taken from quite a few countries, especially Brazil and China, to start programs to control the disease, even in light of the successful story of Japan, that remains the one and only country where schistosomiasis has been eradicated. These programs include sanitation, education, intermediate host control and preventive chemoprophylaxis, alongside of investments into research programs aimed at understanding host-pathogen interactions and at finding new specific drug targets or vaccine candidates. Altogether this world effort might lead to a massive reduction of the worm burden, and possibly (hopefully) to a definitive eradication in the long term.

The present book "Schistosomiasis: epidemiology, diagnosis and treatment" covers a wide range of aspects of such an ancient disease, it is written by healthcare professionals and research specialists in the field, either working in endemic countries or facing with patients coming from endemic areas.

The book is ideally divided into two sections: a first one introducing the basic aspects of the disease, e.g., schistosomes life cycle, the disease's symptoms, the diagnostic tools, the chemotherapy, the control programs; a second one presenting three specific field case studies. The two sections are bridged by one chapter on animal schistosomiasis, showing the threat of infected animals on the disease transmission to humans in endemic areas.

Chapter 1 and 2 explain in details the symptoms, the prophylaxis, the diagnostic tools, the chemotherapeutic tools and the biology of schistosomiasis. These are especially useful to Medical Doctors specializing in tropical medicine and to researchers interested in tropical diseases.

Chapter 3 is focused on chemotherapy and presents a survey of past, present and future drugs for curing the disease in the human host. This is of particular interest to those researchers linking the bench to the bedside, giving them a state-of-the-art of the therapeutic approaches and offering ideas for future directions of drug research.

Chapter 4 is a parallel of chapter 3, but focuses on the interventions to prevent infection of the intermediate snail host and on the research programs aimed at reducing/eliminating this latter. Again this chapter will boost research on the extraction of active principle from plants, cyanobacteria, sponges, able to contrast the expansion of the freshwater snails.

Chapter 5 is focused on animal schistosomiasis in Asia, where this zoonotic disease is particularly pernicious since both livestocks and wild animals act as a reservoir of infections for the human hosts. This subject is quite neglected and is of particular importance for those who are designing intervention programs in endemic areas, where one should take into account not just the human and the snail hosts, but all the human activities around the freshwaters.

Chapter 6 represents the first field case study. Here the authors tackle the incidence of the disease in pre-school children living in endemic areas, who are left aside from the WHO chemoprophylaxis program. The chapter makes a survey of schistosomiasis incidence in this age group in Sub-Saharan Africa, giving the options for an adequate treatment and explaining the challenges of such a program.

Chapter 7 is the second case study. Despite the smaller region surveyed (the Limpopo province, the north-eastern province of South Africa), it clearly shows that women are the most affected in endemic regions. Moreover women with urogenital schistosomiasis are far more susceptible to sexually-transmitted viruses, such as HIV and HPV, and to develop cancer.

Chapter 8 focuses on imported schistosomiasis in Spain, a western country. The authors present the situation of travelers and migrants, with a special focus on children, being all pediatricians.

These last three chapters shed lights into the difficulties and the challenges of large scale preventive programs. Nonetheless they are a useful tool for healthcare managers of both governmental and non-governmental organizations who are going to plan field interventions, which necessarily need a multidisciplinary approach, given the number of factors intervening in the epidemiology of this neglected tropical disease.

This book is meant to mainly target human and veterinary healthcare professionals and medicinal chemistry researchers, therefore it will not cover one branch of schistosomiasis research very recently boosted by the complete sequencing of the genomes of *Schistosoma mansoni*, *S. japonicum* and *S. haematobium*, that investigates on the molecular bases of the disease, by means of genomics, transcriptomics, structural genomics and proteomics. These aspects will be possibly covered by a follow-up.

Finally, I am sure that this book will be an appealing reading and an updating training to medical students and practitioners, independently of their region of intervention, as well as to researchers in basic sciences willing to embrace an exciting applicative field.

Prof. Adriana Erica Miele, PhD
Dept. Biochemical Sciences,
"Sapienza" University of Rome, P.le Aldo Moro 5 00185
Rome, Italy
Tel: +3906 4991 0556
Fax: +3906 444 0062
adriana.miele@uniromal.it

In: Schistosomiasis
Editor: Adriana Erica Miele

ISBN: 978-1-63117-186-4

Chapter 1

The Epidemiology, Pathogenesis, and Clinical Features of Schistosomiasis

Hyasinta Jaka[1*], Anthony Liwa[2] and Phillipo Chalya[3]
[1]Department of Internal Medicine, Bugando Medical Centre and Catholic University of Health and Allied Sciences, Mwanza, Tanzania
[2]Department of Clinical Pharmacology, Catholic University of Health and Allied Sciences, Mwanza, Tanzania
[3]Department of Surgery, Bugando Medical Centre and Catholic University of Health and Allied Sciences, Mwanza, Tanzania

Abstract

Schistosomiasis, sometimes referred to as "bilharziasis", can be associated with serious morbidity and mortality. This chapter fully covers the epidemiology of the disease and the different symptoms and signs.

Chronic complications are generally seen in patients with a high load of parasites. The complications usually occur in individuals who live in endemic areas and who have recurrent exposure. This chapter will also include current updates and the interaction of schistosomes with other

* Corresponding author: Department of Internal Medicine, Bugando Medical Centre and Catholic University of Health and Allied Sciences, PO box 1464, Mwanza, Tanzania. Email: yasintaliwa5@gmail.com.

infections since this is the area of concern to clinicians. Therefore this chapter will be of great value to many clinicians and people who live and/or travel to tropical countries.

Keywords: Life cycle, developmental stages, intermediate hosts, definitive host, pathogenesis, interactions with other infectious diseases

Introduction

There is a number of neglected tropical diseases that cause significant global morbidity in developing countries, including schistosomiasis, trachoma, helminthiasis infections like ascariasis, hookworm, trichuriasis, lymphatic filariasis and onchocerciasis. These diseases affect poor and marginalized communities.

In 1851, Theodor Bilharz detected long worms in the blood of the portal vein during a post-mortem autopsy. Moreover, he discovered strange variations in the mucous membranes of the bladder, seminal glands, ureters, and intestines, as a result of schistosome infection.

Epidemiology

Human schistosomiasis is an incapacitating parasitic disease caused by digenean trematodes of the genus schistosoma; the infection is transmitted through the intermediate snail host. Actually, it is the second common tropical disease after malaria in the world, being endemic in over 70 countries in the tropical areas.

It affects commonly developing countries in Africa, Caribbean, South America, the Middle East and Asia [1], where it is a major source of morbidity and mortality. The number of people treated for schistosomiasis ranged from 12.4 million to 33.5 million between 2006 and 2010. The disease is increasing despite of campaign done by the World Health Organization (WHO). At present about 600 million people are at risk of infection, 200 million people are infected, and the most affected area is the sub-Saharan Africa (SSA).

More than 207 million people in at least 74 counties have active infection and 60% of these have signs and symptoms. Globally, 200,000 deaths are annually caused by schistosomiasis [2, 3]. As a consequence of the chronic infection calcification of the urinary tract, renal failure, cancer of the urinary bladder, periportal fibrosis, and portal hypertension can be rated.

In the places whereby the disease is endemic, the infection is acquired in childhood [4]. In rural areas the transmissions is higher compared to urban areas [5]. The risk of acquiring the disease increases for who live close to the rivers, lakes and rice plantations, while there is no transmission at altitudes of more than 1400 meters from the sea level [6].

Overview of the Species and Life Cycle of Schistosomes

There are about sixteen species of schistosoma, but only five of them cause the infection in human beings (Table 1). They fall under two major groups depending on the outcome of the chronic infection: parasites causing intestinal and hepatic diseases (*S. masoni, S. japonicum, S. mekongi and S. intercalatum*); parasites causing renal and bladder diseases (*S. hematobium*).

The life cycle of all the species of schistosomes is complex (Figure 1), we can distinguish several morphologically and functionally distinct life stages and two phases, based on the type of reproduction: sexual and asexual. Below follows a description of the life stages.

Adult worm: in the final definite host, schistosomes develop up to a pair of female and male worms. The female is permanently hosted in a cavity formed by the body of the adult male, the so called gynechophoric canal. This association is essential for the sexual maturation of the female and, hence, eggs production. The life span is not accurately known, but it is estimated to be more than 30 years [7]. Adult schistosomes belonging to the first group live attached to the walls of the mesenteric periportal veins; those belonging to the second group live attached to the walls of the veins around the bladder.

The eggs: fertilized female schistosomes lay a high number of eggs per day (Table 1), 50% of them pass through the walls of the bladder, or colon to be excreted in urine or faeces, while the others are retained within the tissues, eliciting an inflammation reaction leading to the chronic outcome of the disease.

Miracidium: this form hatches from an egg under favourable conditions (sunlight and temperatures >23°C), uses cilia to swing at 2 mm/s. The miracidium is able to infect snails only for 8-12 h. After penetration, the ciliated surface of the miracidium disappears [8]. The period between the miracidia penetrations to production of cercariae ranges between 4-7 weeks depending on the species, physical environment and other biological factors [9].

Cercaria: it originates from one miracidium after maturation, and it emerges from the snail as free-swimming individual with a tail. In *S. mansoni* and S. *haematobium,* the cercariae production is stimulated by the light and temperature of 10-30 °C, while for *S. japonicum* the production is maximal after the sunset. The life span of cercariae is short: only 36-48 h.

Schistosomulae: once the cercariae have penetrated the human skin (or pharyngeal mucosa) they lose their tails and metamorphose into schistosomula 48hrs after penetration of the subcutaneous tissue, in 5-7days the peak concentration is attained.

Table 1. A summary of the species of schistosomes, the morphology of their eggs, the females eggs production per day and the type of chronic disease

Species	Type of egg spine	Eggs production /day	Disease
S. hematobium	Terminal spine	20-200	Renal and bladder
S. mansoni	Lateral spine	100-300	Intestinal and hepatic
S. japonicum	Rudimentary (oval)	500-35,000	Intestinal
S. intercalatum	Terminal spine	Unknown	Intestinal
S. mekongi	Rudimentary (oval)	Unknown	Intestinal

The sexual phase (humans as the definitive hosts). The human being is infected by free-swimming cercariae, through contact with infected freshwaters. The cercariae develop into schistosomula, which migrate within the vessels to the right side of the lungs uo to the heart, whereby they develop into juvenile worms. These shortly reside in the left side of the heart, and later they migrate to the portal vascular system, where further growth occurs and also pairing of male and female. After a variable period (2-5 weeks post infection) they migrate to the final preferred sites of egg deposition. *S. japonicum* and *S. mekongi* finally reside in the superior and inferior mesenteric veins; while *S. mansoni* and *S. intercalatum* in the inferior mesenteric veins. *S. haematobium* migrates to the vesicle and pelvic plexus after one to three months. This is followed by eggs deposition and excretion. The adult worm pairs can survive for 5-7 years, but they can live up to 30 years [10].

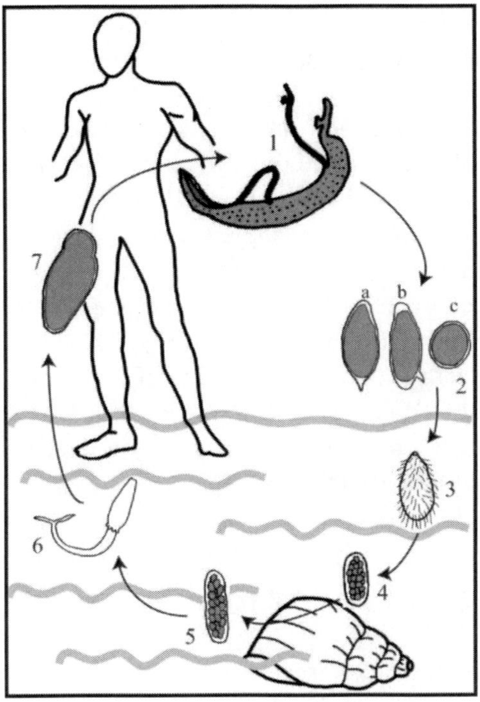

Figure 1. The life cycle of schistosomes, with a morphological description of the different life stages. Adult worms pair (1) living in the definitive human host blood (periportal veins for those species causing intestinal schistosomiasis; peri-bladder veins for those causing urogenital schistosomiasis). Each female lays 20-1000 eggs/day, depending on the species. The eggs (2) are recognizable by their morphology: (a) *S. haematobium* eggs present a terminal spine, (b) *S. mansoni* eggs have a lateral spine; (c) *S. japonicum* eggs are round. The eggs are excreted by either faeces (b,c) or urine (a). Once they reach a freshwater source, they hatch into a free-living ciliated stage called miracidium (3). This one swims towards the mollusc host and penetrates it. Inside the freshwater snails asexual reproduction takes place to increase the number of parasites. Two sequential life stages arise from the miracidium: the mother (4) and the daughter sporocyst (5). This last releases into the water thousands of caudated free living cercariae (6), which are the infective stage for the human host. Cercariae are able to penetrate intact human skin and to develop into a juvenile form: the schistosomulum (7), which migrates undisturbed from the derma to the lungs, where it sexually matures into the adult form (1). This last migrates to the final destination, where it can live for up to 30 years.

As a food source for development, growth and reproduction, schistosomes ingest the host's red blood cells. The ingested red blood cells are lysed inside the oesophagus, while hemoglobin, the main source of amino acids for the worms, is degraded by a complex system of proteases in the gut. The females are more active hence they ingest a larger quantity of red blood cells than males.

The asexual phase (snails as intermediate hosts). The intermediate hosts are freshwater snails, and different worm species can infect different genders of snail (Table 2).

Once excreted in freshwaters the eggs shells rupture and the miracidia hatch. Soon after the miracidia search for a suitable snail host, within 24-48h. Inside the host snail, the miracidium transforms,and for a period of 3-5 weeks undergoes asexual reproduction into sporocysts. Daughter sporocysts migrate in the digestive glands of the snail and each of themt produces thousands of new parasite larvae, the cercariae. The intermediate host snails release about 1500 cercariae every day, four weeks after the infection. Even this free-swimming stage has a short life, maximum 48h.

Pathogenesis and Clinical Features

After penetration, the cercariae shed their tails, change to schistosomula that enter capillaries and lymphatic vessels. Within 12 hours post infection, people may complain about light rash, referred to as "swimmers itch", worse at the area of entrance. Schistosomula will travel in the blood stream to the heart. Through the heart, they migrate to the lung, and after 2-4 weeks they can move to the liver, where they suckle on portal blood, digest red blood cells and undergo rapid growth. Then, the male worm enfold around the female and migrate to the vesicle plexus for *S. haematobium* or to the mesenteric venous plexus for *S. mansoni*, *S. intercalatum* and *S. japonicum*. Each female lays 200 to 2000 eggs each day, starting from the 6th week after penetration. Eggs are shed in the urine (*S. haematobium*) or in the faeces (*S. mansoni, S. intercalatum, S. japonicum*).

The pathology is usually caused largely by schistosome eggs; the adult worms cause little or no lesion to the host unless they migrate to the brain or spinal cord. The adult worms produce cathode and anode associated antigen's these are the antigens which are very important for the diagnosis of schistosomiasis [11].

Table 2. A summary of the gender of snails acting as intermediate hosts to the human schistosome species

Schistosome species	Snails gender
Schistosoma mansoni	Biomphalaria
S. haematobium	Bulinus
S. japonicum	Oncomelania
S. mekongi	Tricula
S. intercalatum	Bulinus

Generally the immunology of schistosomiasis is due to granuloma formation around the tissue-deposited eggs. It is manifested as delayed hypersensitivity through a T-cell mediated immune response from the soluble egg antigens (SEAGs). After the release of the cellular infiltrates found surrounding the eggs, they invade the local tissues and release toxins and enzymes, which initiate immune responses [12, 13]. Schistosomal eggs are surrounded by eosinophils, mononuclear phagocytes, lymphocytes, neutrophils, plasma cells and fibroblasts. The general pathology of schistosomiasis is due to granulomatous lesions which can obstruct vessels and fibro-inflammatory lesions around the trapped eggs [14, 15].

S. hematobium infection. The organs which are affected by *S. hematobium* eggs are the urinary bladder, ureters, vulva, vagina, and cervix [17, 18, 19]. The lesions can present as cancer, polyp, calcification nodules, vesicles ulcers and fibrosis of the bladder [16]. This species only occasionally affects the hepatic tissues.

S. mansoni, S. japonicum, S. mekongi and *S. intercalatum* infection. These parasites' eggs penetrate the bowel through the portal venous system to the hepatic tissue and vessels. In the gut they cause ulceration and scarring [20]. In the liver these eggs are attached in the pre-sinusoidal areas of the portal vein, which blocks the venous blood flow and consequently increases the portal venous pressure. The increase of portal pressure leads to portal hypertension, but there is no hepatocyte dysfunction in periportal fibrosis.

The major cause of clinical disease is the host immune response to the eggs. The worms in the host body tend to coat themselves with hosts antigens, which prevent them from destruction. The eggs produce inflammatory response whereby a host mediated type2 T helper cell (Th2) occurs, which results in activation of fibrosis [21]. The intensity of infection increases between first two decades of life, later it decreases to a very low level [22].

The infection can be asymptomatic, acute or chronic. The acute symptoms tend to be common in population which is non-immune, like for examples travellers. The chronic disease requires a higher load of infection hence occurs in endemic areas. The disease falls under the three groups as follows;

i. *Cercarial dermatitis (swimmers itch), haematuria and diarrhoea*
It is a dermatitis that is caused by penetration of the skin by cercariae. The lesions are post infection pruritic popular rashes in 12-24 hours especially at the site of the larva entry. They can last for up to 7 days or more [5]. After a heavy infection, the early symptoms for *S. haematobium* infection include the detection of blood in the urine (haematuria) [4]. Diarrhoea, with or without blood, is found in infection by *S. mansoni,* but the symptoms are non-specific and very common to other parasitic diseases. In some patients the symptoms of anaemia will appear first, but this common happens in school children.

ii. *Acute schistosomiasis (Katayama fever)*
This is the systemic hypersensitivity reaction against the migrating parasites [4, 22] and occurs 2-8 weeks post infection. This is due to a reaction agkinst the circulating schistosomal antigens. The infected person will present fever, chills, myalgia, arthralgia, dry cough, diarrhoea, headache, lymphadenopathy and hepatosplenomegaly. The infection is nonspecific and disappears as the infection becomes chronic in the body.

iii. *Chronic schistosomiasis infection (and complications)*
It commonly occurs in endemic areas, where the disease severity is directly proportional to the amount of eggs in the tissue, their persistence and distribution [5]. The chronic complications affect the urinary system, hepatic, intestinal, pulmonary, genital and neurological tissues.

Urinary Complications

S. hematobium is the only specie which causes urinary complications. The disease can be either asymptomatic or patients may present haematuria which could be: microscopic haematuria, macroscopic terminal haematuria, throughout haematuria, dysuria and frequency [4]. Patients might also manifest symptoms and signs of anaemia. Each schistosome egg causes an inflammatory response and when the body tries to repair the damage, it causes formation of granuloma lesions. Later on, fibrosis and calcification of the ureters and bladder may occur, which can result in hydroureter and hydronephrosis. This type of schistosomiasis can result into forms of squamous cell carcinoma of the bladder [23], and immune complex deposition in the kidneys which lead to massive proteinuria and consequently nephrotic syndrome [24].

Intestinal and Hepatic Complications

Hepatic diseases occur with *S. mansoni*, *S. japonicum* and *S. mekongi* infections. Patients may have abdominal pain, blood in stool, poor appetite and diarrhoea. Colitis, hepatomegaly and severe splenomegaly do occur in children and adolescents in endemic areas. Symmer's pipestem fibrosis is the diffuse deposition of the collagens/granuloma formation in the periportal spaces due to egg deposition. This increases the portal pressure and results into portal hypertension and increased splenomegaly. The portal vein carries about 1500 ml/min of blood from the bowel, spleen, and stomach to the liver at a pressure of 5-10 mmHg. Any obstruction or increased resistance to this flow as well as pathological increases in portal blood flow may lead to portal hypertension with portal pressures over 12 mmHg. Increases in portal pressure cause development of a porto-systemic collateral circulation with resultant compensatory porto-systemic shunting and disturbed intrahepatic circulation. The patients with portal hypertension may present with oesophageal varices with or without hematemesis (Figure 2), haemorrhoids, signs of anaemia and ascites.

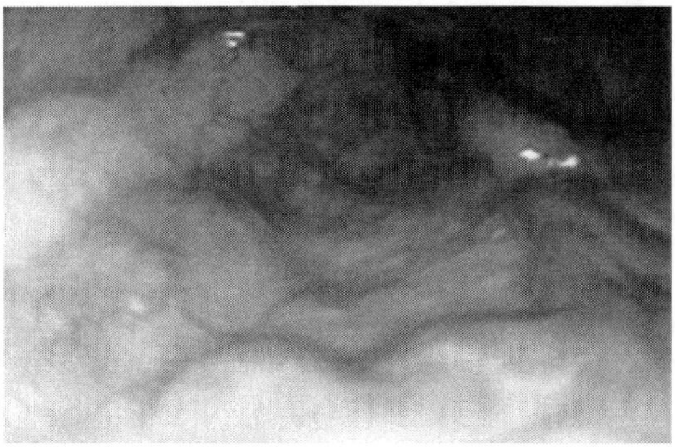

Figure 2. Oesophageal varicess due to portal hypertension caused by schistosomiasis.

Neurologic Complications (Neuroschistosomiasis)

Adult worm may migrate to either the spinal cord or the brain, and sometimes the eggs may enter the vertebral venous plexus, consequently embedding into the spinal cord or the brain and resulting in granulomas at these sites. Neurological symptoms result from the inflammatory reaction of the host to eggs deposited in these sites.

Eggs in the spinal cord

The prevalence of oviposition in the spinal cord ranges from 0.3% to 13%. It can present symptoms common to myelopathy (acute transverse myelitis and subacute myeloradiculopathy). This does occur early after infection, whereby Patients usually refer rapidly progressing lower limb pain, weakness and bowel dysfunction, the thoracolumbar region of the spinal cord is most frequently reported [25, 26]. The conus medullaris and cauda equina are the most common sites of involvement. Myelopathy can provoke a complete flaccid paraplegia with areflexia, sphincter dysfunction and sensory disturbances.

Eggs in the brain

Eggs deposition in the brain can provoke localised lesions in the cerebellar or cerebrum, which result into focal CNS impairment, increased intracranial pressure and seizures [27, 28]. In the cerebral schistosomiasis, loss of consciousness, seizures, delirium dysphasia, focal motor deficits, ataxia and visual field impairment are numbered within the symptoms. Sometimes, cerebral and cerebellar tumour-like symptoms can appear such as increased intracranial pressure, headache, nausea and vomiting.

Pulmonary Complications

When there is heavy infection with *S. mansoni*, *S. japonicum* or *S. haematobium*, eggs from the portal circulation can penetrate into the pulmonary circulation and produce a granulomatous pulmonary endarteritis [29]. This results into portal-pulmonary hypertension and consequently cor pulmonale (right sided heart failure secondary to lung diseases) due to increase in pulmonary resistance. Cor pulmonale has commonly a chronic and slowly progressive course. The patient may complain of exceptional dyspnoea tachypnea, fatigue and cough. Angina-like chest pain, which does not respond to nitrates, can also occur and may be due to right ventricular ischemia. Hemoptysis may occur because of rupture of a dilated or fibrotic pulmonary artery and signs of right heart failure with systemic venous congestion, like left parasternal or subxiphoid heave, hepato-jugular reflux and pulsatile liver, may occur. Post chemotherapy, the adult worms may reside into the lungs and cause coughing, wheezing, dyspnoea, and can be visible as pulmonary infiltrates on X-rays [30].

Genital Complications

In urinary schistosomiasis, vulvar hypertrophy and ulcerations are common, and also vagina and cervical ulcerations can occur [4, 31]. Infertility can be a consequence if either ovaries or fallopian tubes are involved in females; while the spermatic chord, testicles, epididymis or even prostate can be involved in men in endemic areas.

Relationship of Schistosomiasis with other Infectious Diseases

i) Association with Salmonelosis

Salmonella typhi and *S. paratyphi* tend to attach to the tegument or in the gut of the adult schistosome, when they ingest bacteria and, hence they serve as a reservoir for infections. They can also enter the bloodstream from areas of inflamed GI mucosa that has been damaged by the eggs. Salmonella association to Schistosoma is mediated by pili which recognize and associate with glycolipids receptors on the surface of schistosomes [32, 33].

ii) HIV Infection

HIV affects schistosomiasis. The IgE and eosinophils may play an important role in protecting the host against schistosomes. In endemic areas people do acquire some form of immunity after years of exposure, which is mediated by IgE. Immune response and eosinophilic expression can be affected by HIV disease, which could result into increased susceptibility to reinfection with schistosomes [34,35]. HIV patients with low CD4+ T-cell counts may have an increased susceptibility to schistosomes infection and egg excretion. Moreover, immune restoration syndrome in one HIV patient, also affected by schistosomiasis, and receiving antiretroviral therapy has been observed [36].

Schistosomiasis affects HIV infection. Mucosal damage in the genitalia is the one of the risk factor for HIV transmission. In fact the eggs of *S. hematiobium* induce inflammation in the lower reproductive tract, especially in females, therefore this increases the risk of HIV transmission [37, 38]. HIV co-infected schistosomiasis patients have also been reported to have faster progression of the AIDS disease [39]. In schistosome infected patients, who are HIV-seropositive, interference with host immune response is reported, therefore determining increased HIV replication and cytokine dysregulation.

iii) Viral Hepatitis

When there is co-infections of schistosomiasis and viral hepatitis B or C, the disease has more severe outcome and a worse prognosis than those infected with only one pathogen [40, 41]. Alteration of cellular immunity, increase in viral RNA content together with increased risk of chronicity occurs in patients with hepatitis C infection, when co-infected with schistosomes [42].

References

[1] Schistosomiasis, facts sheet No 115 February 2010: World health organisation. Available at http://www.who.int/mediacentre/facesheets/fs115/en/index.html.

[2] King, CH. Toward the elimination of schistosomiasis. *N Engl J Med*, 2009, 360(2), 106-9.

[3] Chistulo, L; Loverde, P; Engels, D. Disease Watch: Schistosomiasis. *TDR Nature Reviews Microbiology*, 2004, 2, 12.

[4] Gryseels, B; Polman, K; Clerinx, J; Kestens, L. Human schistosomiasis. *Lancet*, 2006, 368, 1106.

[5] Lucey, DR; Maguire, JH. Schistosomiasis. *Infect Dis Clin North Am*, 1993, 7, 635.

[6] Kabatereine, NB; Brooker, S; Tukahebwa, EM; et al. Epidemiology and geography of Schistosoma mansoni in Uganda: implications for planning control. *Trop Med Int Health*, 2004, 9, 372.
[7] Chabasse, D; Bertrand, G; Leroux, JP; et al. Bilhaziaose a *Schistosoma mansoni* evolutive decouverte 37ans après l'infection. *Bull Soc Pathol Exot filiales*, 1985, 78, 643-647
[8] Jourdane, J; Theron, A. Larval development; eggy to cercariae. In Rollinson D & Simpson AJ (eds). *The biology of Schistosomiasis*: from Genes to Latrines. London: Academic Press, 1987, 83-113.
[9] Webbe, G. The life cycle of the parasites. In Jordan P & Webbe G (eds) *Schistosomiasis, Epidemiology, Treatment and control*, London: Heinemann, 1982, 50-78.
[10] Arnon, R. *Life span of parasite in schistosomiasis patients. Isr J Med Sci*, 1990, 26, 404.
[11] De Jonge, N; Gryseel, B; Hilberath, GW; et al. Detection of circulating anodic antigen by ELISA for seroepidemiology of schistosomiasis mansoni. *Trans R Soc Trop eMed Hyg*, 1988, 82, 591-594.
[12] Keating, JH; Wilson, RA; Skelly, PJ. No overt cellular inflammation around intravascular schistosomes in vivo. *J Parasitol*, 2006, 92, 1365.
[13] Coutinho, HM; Acosta, LP; Wu, HW; et al. Th2 cytokines are associated with persistent hepatic fibrosis in human *Schistosoma japonicum* infection. *J Infect Dis*, 2007, 195, 288.
[14] Von Lichtenberg, E. Consequences of infection with schistosomes. In Rollinson D & Simpson AJG (eds). *The biology of schistosomiasis: from Genes to Latrines*. London: Academic Press, 1987, 185-232.
[15] Cheever, AW; Hoffmann, KF; Wynn, TA. Immunopathology of schistosomiasis mansoni in mice and men. *Immunol Today*, 2000, 21, 465.
[16] Smith, JH; Kamel, IA; Elwi, A; Kamel, IA; et al. A quantitative post mortem analysis of urinary schistosomiasis in Egypt. I. Evolution and epidemiology. *Am J Trop Med Hyg*, 1974, 23, 1054-1071.
[17] Smith, JH; Kamel, IA; Elwi, A; et al. A quantitative post mortem analysis of urinary schistosomiasis in Egypt. II. Evolution and epidemiology. *Am J Trop Med Hyg*, 1975, 24, 806-822.
[18] Downs, JA; Kabangila Verweij, JJ; Jaka, H; et al. Detectable urogenital schistosome DNA and cervical abnormalities 6 months after single-dose Praziquantel in women with Schistosoma haematobium infection. *Trop Med Int Health*, 2013.

[19] Strickland, GT. Gastrointestinal manifestations of schistosomiasis. *Gut*, 1994, 35, 133.

[20] Bartley, PB; Ramm, GA; Jones, MK; et al. A contributory role for activated hepatic stellate cells in the dynamics of *Schistosoma japonicum* egg-induced fibrosis. *Int J Parasitol*, 2006, 36, 993.

[21] Butterworth, AE. Immunological aspects of human schistosomiasis. *Br Med Bull*, 1998, 54, 357.

[22] Ross, AG; Vickers, D; Olds, GR; et al. Katayama syndrome. *Lancet Infect Dis*, 2007, 7, 218.

[23] Ross, AG; Bartley, PB; Sleigh, AC; et al. Schistosomiasis. *N Engl J Med*, 2002, 346, 1212.

[24] Andrade, ZA; Rocha, H. Schistosomal glomerulopathy. *Kidney Int*, 1979, 16, 23.

[25] Ferrari, TC. Involvement of central nervous system in the schistosomiasis. *Mem Inst Oswaldo Cruz*, 2004, 99, 59.

[26] Ferrari, TC. Spinal cord schistosomiasis. A report of 2 cases and review emphasizing clinical aspects. *Medicine (Baltimore)*, 1999, 78, 176.

[27] Nascimento-Carvalho, CM; Moreno-Carvalho, OA. Neuroschistosomiasis due to *Schistosoma mansoni:* a review of pathogenesis, clinical syndromes and diagnostic approaches. *Rev Inst Med Trop Sao Paulo*, 2005, 47, 179.

[28] Kim, AH; Maher, CO; Smith, ER. Lumbar intramedullary spinal schistosomiasis presenting as progressive paraparesis: case report. *Neurosurgery*, 2006, 58, E996; discussion E996.

[29] Andrade, ZA; Andrade, SG. Pathogenesis of schistosomal pulmonary arteritis. *Am J Trop Med Hyg*, 1970, 19, 305.

[30] Pedroso, ER; Lambertucci, JR; Greco, DB; et al. Pulmonary schistosomiasis mansoni: post-treatment pulmonary clinical-radiological alterations in patients in the chronic phase: a double-blind study. *Trans R Soc Trop Med Hyg*, 1987, 81, 778.

[31] Chen, W; Flynn, EA; Shreefter, MJ; Blagg, NA. Schistosomiasis: an unusual finding of the cervix. *Obstet Gynecol*, 2012, 119, 472.

[32] Elliott, DE. Schistosomiasis. Pathophysiology, diagnosis, and treatment. *Gastroenterol Clin North Am*, 1996, 25, 599.

[33] Melhem, RF; Loverde, PT. AMechanism of interaction of salmonella and Schistosoma species. *Infect Immun*, 1984, 44(2), 274-281.

[34] Joseph, S; Jones, FM; Laidlaw, ME; et al. Impairment of the *Schistosoma mansoni*-specific immune responses elicited by treatment

with praziquantel in Ugandans with HIV-1 coinfection. *J Infect Dis*, 2004, 190, 613.

[35] Ganley-Leal, LM; Mwinzi, PN; Cetre-Sossah, CB; et al. Correlation between eosinophils and protection against reinfection with *Schistosoma mansoni* and the effect of human immunodeficiency virus type 1 coinfection in humans. *Infect Immun*, 2006, 74, 2169.

[36] de Silva, S; Walsh, J; Brown, M. Symptomatic *Schistosoma mansoni* infection as an immune restoration phenomenon in a patient receiving antiretroviral therapy. *Clin Infect Dis*, 2006, 42, 303.

[37] Feldmeier, H; Krantz, I; Poggensee, G. Female genital schistosomiasis as a risk-factor for the transmission of HIV. *Int J STD AIDS*, 1994, 5, 368.

[38] Downs, JA; Dam, GJ; Changalucha, JM; et al. Association of Schistosomiasis and HIV Infection in Tanzania. *Am J. Trop. Med. Hyg*. 2012, 87(5), 868-873

[39] Mbabazi, PS; Andan, O; Fitzgerald, DW; Chitsulo, L; Engels, D; Downs, JA. Examining the relationship between urogenital schistosomiasis and HIV infection. *PloS Negl Trop Dis*, 2011.

[40] Lambertucci, JR; Rayes, AA; Serufo, JC; et al. Schistosomiasis and associated infections. *Mem Inst Oswaldo Cruz*, 1998, 93 Suppl 1, 135.

[41] Strickland, GT. Liver disease in Egypt: hepatitis C superseded schistosomiasis as a result of iatrogenic and biological factors. *Hepatology*, 2006, 43, 915.

[42] Kamal, SM; Turner, B; He, Q; et al. Progression of fibrosis in hepatitis C with and without schistosomiasis: correlation with serum markers of fibrosis. *Hepatology*, 2006, 43,771.

In: Schistosomiasis
Editor: Adriana Erica Miele
ISBN: 978-1-63117-186-4

Chapter 2

The Diagnosis, Treatment Options and Prevention of Schistosomiasis

Hyasinta Jaka[1*] and Anthony Liwa[2]
[1]Department of Internal Medicine, Bugando Medical Centre and Catholic University of Health and Allied Sciences, Mwanza, Tanzania
[2]Department of Clinical Pharmacology, Catholic University of Health and Allied Sciences, Mwanza, Tanzania

Abstract

Schistosomiasis or "Bilharzia" is a tropical parasitic disease associated with serious morbidity and mortality. This chapter fully covers schistosomiasis management, which includes the diagnosis, treatment options, and prevention of the parasitic disease.

This chapter includes current methods of early diagnosis of schistosomiasis, outlines the treatments options and will help many clinicians in properly managing their patients.

* Corresponding author: Department of Internal Medicine, Bugando Medical Centre and Catholic University of Health and Allied Sciences, PO box 1464, Mwanza, Tanzania. Email: yasintaliwa@gmail.com.

Keywords: Microscopic diagnosis, serological tests, ELISA, PCR, therapy, prophylaxis

Introduction

Schistosomiasis is one of the most prevalent parasitic diseases. It is estimated that more than 10% of the world's population is at risk and more than 207 million people in at least 74 countries have active infection and 60% of these have signs and symptoms.

The causative agent of schistosomiasis is a trematode worm of the genus Schistosoma. There are three main species that parasitize humans: *S. haematobium*, *S. japonicum,* and *S. mansoni*. Other species with more localized regional spectrum include: *S. intercalatum S. mekongi* as well as *S. malayensis*.

The highest prevalence of schistosomiasis is usually seen in school-age children and adolescents, where it represents the main cause of iron deficiency and anemia, hence poor growth and poor class concentration. It is known that Schistosomiasis-related complications are underestimated. The diagnosis is done in symptomatic and asymptomatic people who are suspected to be at risk. Most of the schistosomiasis infected people may remain not symptomatic for a long period.

Microscopic identification of eggs in stools and urine, or in tissue, is one of the ways of arriving at a positive diagnosis. Current diagnosis involves detection of parasitic antigens by enzyme-linked immunosorbent assay (ELISA) tests methods; in equipped Hospitals and analytical laboratories the Polymerase Chain Reaction (PCR) can also be done. Serology detection can be useful in both clinical management and for epidemiologic surveys. In general full range of blood tests can be done to detect anaemia, renal function, liver enzymes, and many other blood related complications. Imaging Studies and endoscopies can help in certain stages of the disease development, especially when there are complications.

Drugs like Praziquantel have been and are in use to treat schistosomiasis, together with very few other drugs, which will be discussed. There is a number of factors, which have contributed to the use of Praziquantel, like its excellent pharmacological properties, its effectiveness after one dose, the lack of toxicity, its low cost, and its high shelf-life.

Diagnosis of Schistosomiasis

Blood Tests

These tests are sometimes useful in evaluating the severity of schistosomal infection, and also in assisting the diagnosis.

Serology

Seroconversion generally occurs 4 to8 weeks after infection. Antibodies usually detected are the antischistosomal antibodies in serum samples of patients. These antibodies are directed against extracts of adult worm's egg or cercariae. These can be tested in a patient from a non-endemic areas. However, they cannot differentiate the active from past infestations, neither they can quantify the eggs burden. The detection of antibodies against *S. mansoni* adult worm microsomal antigen (MAMA), *S. haematobium* and *S. japonicum* adult worm microsomal antigens (JAMA) has been reported to be highly specific for those three species. Nevertheless their presence needs to be confirmed by ELISA first and then by Western Blot techniques The specificity and sensitivity of the ELISA tests against MAMA and JAMA is reported to be higher than 90% and 95%, respectively [1].

The presence of antigens reflects infection in a patient, but this can be detected in *urine or serum*. There are two gut-associated parasite proteins: circulating cathodic antigen (CCA) and circulating anodic antigen (CAA), which are present in the blood when there is active infection or current infection [1-3]. These tests can be used to assess treatment efficacy in patients under cure, where the absence of circulating antigens indicates clearance from the adult worms. Studies have shown that, antigen tests may become negative as early as 5 to 10 days after treatment.

Polymerase chain reaction assays

PCR assays are being developed for the diagnosis of schistosomiasis. The real time quantitative PCR is more sensitive than classic diagnosis tools based on microscopy and serology [1-5]. This is the current methods of early diagnosis of schistosomiasis. Antigen and PCR assay–based testing can always confirm a diagnosis.

Complete blood count

The routine full blood count will show eosinophilia, especially during the acute phase. Eosinophilia depends on the duration, stage and intensity of the infection together with genetic makeup of an individual [2, 6, 7]. Moreover, from this analysis anaemia can be highlighted, due to blood loss.

Liver tests

In case of hepatic granulomatosis, there will be an increased alkaline phosphatase level and gamma-glutamyltransferase (GGT) level leaving the transaminases unaffected.

Renal function

Renal functionality tests can be requested in case of severe obstructive nephropathy, which causes the renal function to decline.

Blood culture

Sometimes the blood cultures may be indicated for persons, who may have developed recurrent salmonella infections with severe schistosomiasis and patients with persistent or recurrent fevers.

Microscopic Examination of Schistosoma Eggs

Identification of parasite eggs in tissue, stool or urine by microscope is one of the reference methods of diagnosis of schistosomiasis. This method can identify the type of species. Indeed, the eggs have different spines, which can be seen on microscopy and which usually differentiates these species (see also Chapter 1 in this book). The eggs of *S. haematobium* have a terminal spine, *S. japonicum* eggs are spheroidal with a small knob and *S. mansoni* eggs have a lateral spine.

Urinary microbiology

Wherever there is either macroscopic or microscopic haematuria (detected by urine dipsticks), it is most likely to be positive for *S hematobium*. The study done by Harries and others found that 78% of British expatriates with eggs in their urine had positive hematuria on dipstick [8]. Detection of *S. haematobium* will be enhanced by centrifugation and examination of the sediment under a microscope. Quantification is possible by using filtration method through a nucleopore membrane of a given standard volume of urine followed by egg counts.

Fecal microbiology

Concentration methods can be used in case of a very light infestation to enhance eggs detection such as the formalin-ethyl acetate technique. It is done on thick smears to detect Schistosomiasis with primary bowel infection, but frank blood or heme can also be detected.

During field surveys, the eggs output can be quantified by using the Kato-Katz technique on about 20 to 50 mg of faecal material or the Ritchie technique. These techniques are useful to show the number of eggs excreted per day.

In some laboratories, morphologic details and staining can detect solitary and mixed schistosomal species in each infected individual.

Tissue biopsy

Sigmoidoscopy/proctoscopy or cystoscopy can be done to take biopsy from rectal and urinary bladder, which may show eggs when stool or urine examinations are negative, but pedunculated and sessile polyps can also be identified. Other tissue sites where the eggs can be detected are specimens of pulmonary, liver and cervical tissues [3, 8-11].

Egg viability test

Viability testing requires mixing the stools or urine with distilled water and observing for hatching miracidia at room temperature. Whenever the infection is active, viable eggs are produced, while old infections or treated patients result in nonviable eggs and absence of miracidia.

Investigations during complications

Radiology and imaging techniques

These include the plain abdominal radiography to detect calcifications, intravenous pyelography for bladder, ureter changes, obstructive uropathy. In addition, computer tomography can detect renal and brain lesions [12]. Chest radiographs may show patchy infiltrates in acute schistosomiasis and pulmonary hypertension in late stages, even cor pulmonale can be demonstrated.

Myelography can detect suspected spinal cord damage and portal pressure, while portal venography can be used to detect the portal venous hypertensive changes.

Ultrasonography can also be used to identify organ enlargements, like ureters (hydronephrosis), liver, spleen. In complicated schistosomiasis this diagnostic tool detects periportal fibrosis and ascites in portal hypertension. This is a more important predictor of morbidity and mortality than Child-Pugh score. The Doppler ultrasonography is non-invasive evaluation used in assessment of severity of portal hypertension and vasoactive drug response in patients with portal hypertension and bleeding varices [13]. The echocardiography can show pulmonary hypertension and cor pulmonale. The use of computed tomography (CT) and magnetic resonance imaging (MRI) scanning may be useful in diagnosing either central nervous system involvement or periportal fibrosis. In the brain it may show ring-enhancing lesions surrounding edema and in the spinal cord (through the Batson plexus) it will highlight granulomatous lesions of the conus medularis and cauda equine.

Other Procedures

Upper gastrointestinal endoscopy can detect oesophageal varices; it can also be used for treating the bleeding due to ruptured oesophageal and gastric varices.

Management of Schistosomiasis

The treatment depends on the stage of the disease, whether the patient had presented with acute, chronic infections or with complications. There are groups of patients who will receive the chemotherapy, and other groups of patients that will get management of complications first, depending on the severity of area affected and on the type of syndromes they have.

Chemotherapy

The aim of the chemotherapy is the cure of the patient by eliminating the infection, this leads to cessation of eggs deposition, prevents further tissue damage and regression of the existing lesions. The assessment of the chemotherapy should be done to patients treated for schistosomiasis. This can be done by clinical improvement, through urine or stool specimen analysis, from at least six weeks post treatment in endemic areas, but three months in non-endemic areas. Moreover, the assessment can be done by radiological signs, for example the ultrasonography and endoscopy. The serology is not recommended since it remains positive for prolonged time following therapy.

The different types of medications used in schistosomiasis

In the 1970s, Pfizer, in England, produced oxamniquine and Merck, in Germany, produced praziquantel (PZQ). These drugs were shown to have a high curative power against schistosomiasis, when used orally in a single dose, or as a series of two doses. Additionally, they showed fewer side effects. Thus, they conformed to the standards for ideal drugs proposed by the World Health Organization (WHO). These drugs have been extremely important for treating individuals with schistosomiasis, both for short-term prevalence control and for medium to long-term morbidity control [14].

Praziquantel

PZQ is a highly effective commercially readily available drug. So far, no backup compound for PZQ of comparable efficacy and breadth of application is available [15]. PZQ [2-(cyclohexylcarbonyl) x1,2,3,6,7,11b-hexahydro- 4H-pyrazino [2,1-a]isoquinoline-4-one] is a bitter-tasting white crystalline powder. It is normally stable, practically insoluble in water and soluble in some organic solvents. It is usually a racemate mixture composed of equal parts of 'laevo' and 'dextro' isomers, of which only the former is schistosomicidally active either in vivo or in vitro. Tablets of PZQ usually contain 600 mg of active ingredient. A syrup formulation containing 600 mg/5 ml suitable for small children is available from some manufacturers: e.g., Epiquantel, which is produced in Egypt [16].

Mode of action of PZQ

PZQ is a broad-spectrum anthelmintic active against schistosome species which are major parasites of man. Two major effects on *S. mansoni* have been demonstrated: (i) spastic paralysis of the parasite musculature, possibly arising as a consequence of an influx of Ca^{2+} into the worm and (ii) vacuolation and degeneration of the worm. Recent work indicates the beta (β) subunits of voltage-gated calcium ions (Ca^{2+}) channels are the molecular targets of PZQ [17-18], although still a few controversies remain [19]. Damage caused by

PZQ increases exposure of antigens on the worm surface, particularly over male worm tubercles and this in turn seemingly renders the worms more susceptible to antibody attack [18]. This drug-induced antigen exposure is assumed to account for the synergistic effect between PZQ and host antibodies in killing the worms *in vivo* [20].

Pharmacokinetics of PZQ

Absorption is considered to be good at 75 to100% of an oral dose in man; the maximum concentration (tmax) is reached after 30 to 120 minutes in animals and up to 3 to 4 hours in humans. There is considerable inter-individual variation for unknown reasons in the rate of absorption and clearance, so maximum concentration (Cmax), tmax and area under the concentration curve (AUC) show wide ranges. A carbohydrate-rich meal enhances absorption in man. Co-administration of Chloroquine and pre-administration of Carbamazepine and Phenytoin may reduce the bioavailability of PZQ. There is an extensive first pass metabolism of PZQ in all animals in the liver to mono- and dihydroxylated derivatives, many of which are conjugated. A few of the metabolites possess some but weaker anti-parasitic activity, therefore PZQ itself is the important therapeutic agent.

Overall clearance is rapid, with a half-life ($t_{1/2}$) of unchanged PZQ of 1-2 hours in most species and of metabolites of 3-8 hours. Clearance of metabolites, which is limited by the rate of metabolism, is slower and metabolites are completely cleared by 4 days after one oral dose. PZQ is 80% bound to plasma proteins.

PZQ is excreted as metabolites, although some parent drug may be detected in urine. Metabolites in urine accounted for 38 and 66% of an oral dose in rat and dog, respectively, within 8 hours and about 15% in bile. In human about 80% of a dose is excreted in urine. PZQ and its principal metabolites are found in human milk at levels about 25% of those in plasma and following the same rapid time course.

First pass metabolism in the liver is rapid: 15 minutes after one oral dose. PZQ is metabolized to mono-, di- and tri-hydroxylated compounds by CYP1A2, CYP3A4 and CYP2C19 in human liver microsomes. The metabolite found in a higher proportion in human serum is trans-4-hydroxypraziquantel (4-OHPZQ). The enzyme(s) responsible has not been definitely identified, but it is likely at least to include a member of the P450 3A4 family in lamb and rat, judged by selective inhibition experiments [21].

Efficacy and Dose of PZQ

PZQ is the active agent against the adult stages of schistosomes. Thus, the main limitation to its use is the lack of therapeutic efficacy against early stages. This could be the main reason for the many treatment failures observed and high rates of re-infection [22].

The World Health Organization (WHO) currently recommends that it should be used in one single dose of 40 mg/kg for the treatment of both urinary and intestinal schistosomiasis, different doses of PZQ are being deployed by national control programmes [23]. In order to eradicate any surviving schistosomes, a second course of PZQ after two to three months is also required.

Alternative Therapies

Oxamniquine

This is a 2-aminomethyltetrahydroquinoline derivative, it is produced by biological synthesis and it was one of the most promising schistosomicides. It has an anticholinergic effect, which increases the parasite's motility and inhibits nucleic acid synthesis. It is more effective against male than female parasites and it is effective only against *S. mansoni*. It is ineffective against *S. haematobium, S. japonicum* or other schistosome species that parasitize humans [23].

This drug was distributed as 250 mg capsules or in suspensions of 250 mg per 5 ml. The mechanism of action for Oxamniquine was characterised by an early inhibition of oviposition by the females and by the presence of tegumental lesions on worms moving to the liver, where they were then phagocytized [14]. In contrast to PZQ, the mechanism of action of oxamniquine is relatively well understood: it has to be activated by a parasite sulfotransferase, in fact resistant/insusceptible schistosomes lack the enzymatic activity. Moreover, in contrast to PZQ, the price of oxamniquine has remained high and for this reason alone it is unlikely to be much used in Africa. So far its use has been almost entirely restricted to Brazil and other South American countries. Its use was, however, quite extensive: over 12 million doses were administered in Brazil in a schistosomiasis control organized by that country's Ministry of Health. Oxamniquine may be particularly prone to the problem of drug-resistance but it may be needed because it is effective against *S. mansoni* infections in an area in which PZQ gave poor cure rates [16].

Artemisinin and its Derivatives

Artemisinin, the active ingredient of the plant *Artemisia annua*, is a sesquiterpene lactone from which semi-synthetic derivatives have been synthesized, including artemether and artesunate. These are potent anti-malaria drugs and millions of doses have been administered for this purpose. Artemisinin activity against *S. japonicum* was discovered in the early 1980s and *in vivo* activity against other schistosome species confirmed subsequently. These compounds are well tolerated and give no or only mild side effects, but their mechanisms of action are not yet fully understood.

Artemisinins are of particular interest because, in contrast to PZQ and Oxamniquine, they show highest activity against immature worms. Artemether and Artesunate have therefore been used in China as ‘prophylactics’ against *S. japonicum* infection during major floods and their chemoprophylactic effectiveness has also been demonstrated in Africa against both *S. mansoni* and *S. haematobium.* They may be particularly useful in areas with high rates of infection transmission and where PZQ is less effective, perhaps because of the insensitivity of immature schistosomes to the latter [16]. However, several reviews have suggested that artemisinin derivatives exert only a moderate degree of efficacy against Schistosomiasis. Meanwhile, artemisinin derivatives have been used in successfully combination with other compounds for the treatment of malaria, reducing the probability of selecting drug-resistant parasites. Moreover, synthetic artemisins (e.g., trioxolanes) are also active against juvenile and adult schistosomes but no schistosome-specific clinical trials with synthetic artemisinins have been undertaken so far [22].

Management of Different Syndromes

Katayama fever

PZQ is not effective at this stage, and treatment regimen for Katayama syndrome is not known, it is mostly supportive. Glucocorticoids (for example prednisolone 40 mg daily for five days) can be used to relief symptoms. The first dose of PZQ should be administered within 6 to 10 weeks, in the dose of 40 mg/kg. In order to eradicate any surviving schistosomes, a second course of PZQ after two to three months is also required.

Neurological schistosomiasis

When the disease involves the Central nervous system (CNS), PZQ together with glucocorticoids should be given. When a patient presents with convulsion, anticonvulsants should be given.

Portal hypertension

Portal hypertension can complicate to oesophageal varices, and this condition can be managed by either primary prophylaxis (when there is no upper gastrointestinal Bleeding) or secondary prophylaxis when (the patient had already bled). PZQ dose should be given in all patients with varices. Primary prophylaxis is achieved by endoscopic variceal banding ligation (EVBL) and non-selective beta blockers, or non-selective beta blockers alone in areas where there is no EVBL. In any case the non-selective beta blockers do not prevent varices. The secondary prophylaxis includes EVBL, non-selective beta blockers, with either splenectomy or transjugular intra hepatic portal systemic shunts (TIPS), in case of a failure of the first one.

Schistosomiasis with other infections

The response to antibiotics is good, but recurrence is common unless the underlying Schistosomiasisis is managed, to prevent further relapses of bacterial infection. In fact eradication of the adult worms is recommended. Studies have shown that the efficacy of antibiotics, which are commonly used to treat salmonella, decreased by factor of 4-16 folds due to this association [25].

Schistosomiasis in Pregnancy and lactating mothers

Pregnant women were usually excluded from treatment campaigns of Schistosomiasis. Studies have shown that, there is no increase in the rate of preterm deliveries, abortion or congenital defects when compared with untreated women [26]. Also there were no teratogenic effects after one single oral 40 mg/kg dose of PZQ, neither stillbirths nor congenital abnormalities in the babies, who were followed for one year later after birth, were reported [27-28]. Hence, since 2003 WHO prescribed that pregnant and lactating women in Schistosomiasis endemic areas should not be excluded from receiving treatment with PZQ [29], while pregnant mothers should be given PZQ only after the first trimester.

Prevention and Control of Schistosomiasis

Prevention

Infection by Schistosomes can be prevented by avoiding swimming or wading in freshwater, which are at high risk. The water for drinking should be boiled, and the bathing water should settle for one to two days before use. Sanitation is a must in order to prevent urines and faeces to get in contact with freshwaters.

Control

The control of Schistosomiasis is focusing on the following points: (i) the reduction of the number of infected people by early diagnosis and mass treatment; (ii) elimination of the snails by molluscides.

Control interventions targeted towards schistosomiasis, as presently recommended by WHO, have as primary focus the provision of free treatment with PZQ to school-aged children (SAC), 5–14 years old, as well as, adults (≥15 years old), who reside within disease endemic regions [25]. The environmental control of snail breeding sites has been tried, snails repopulation occurs rapidly and so eradication is difficult to sustain. Clinical screening is the option for people moved from endemic area, because the disease can remain asymptomatic for a long time.

References

[1] Sandoval, N; Siles-Lucas, M; Pérez-Arellano, JL; Carranza, C; Puente, S; López-Abán, J; Muro, A. A new PCR-based approach for the specific amplification of DNA from different Schistosoma species applicable to human urine samples. *Parasitology*, 2006, 133(Pt 5), 581-587.

[2] Gundersen, SG; Ravn, J; Haagensen, I. Early detection of circulating anodic antigen (CAA) in a case of acute schistosomiasis mansoni with Katayama fever. *Scand J Infect Dis*, 1992, 24, 549-552.

[3] Deelder, AM; Qian, ZL; Kremsner, PG; Acosta, L; Rabello, AL; Enyong, P; Simarro, PP; van Etten, EC; Krijger, FW; Rotmans, JP; et al. Quantitative diagnosis of Schistosoma infections by measurement of

circulating antigens in serum and urine. *Trop Geogr Med*, 1994, 46, 233-238.

[4] Downs, JA; Kabangila Verweij, JJ; Jaka, H; Peck, RN; Kalluvya, SE; Changalucha, JM; Johnson, WD; van Lieshout, L; Fitzgerald, DW. Detectable urogenital schistosome DNA and cervical abnormalities 6 months after single-dose praziquantel in women with Schistosoma haematobium infection. *Trop Med Int Health*, 2013, 18(9),1090-1096.

[5] Wichmann, D; Poppert, S; Von Thien, H; Clerinx, J; Dieckmann, S; Jensenius, M; Parola, P; Richter, J; Schunk, M; Stich, A; Zanger, P; Burchard, GD; Tannich, E. Prospective European-wide multicenter study on a blood based real-time PCR for the diagnosis of acute Schistosomiasis. *BMC Infect*, 2013, 13, 55.

[6] Pardo, J; Carranza, C; Muro, A; Angel-Moreno, A; Martín, AM; Martín, T; Hernández-Cabrera, M; Pérez-Arellano, JL. Helminth-related Eosinophilia in African immigrants, Gran Canaria. *Emerg Infect Dis.*, 2006 Oct, 12(10), 1587-1589.

[7] Mahmoud, AA. The ecology of eosinophils in schistosomiasis. *J Infect Dis*, 1982, 145, 613-622.

[8] Harries, AD; Fryatt, R; Walker, J; Chiodini, PL; Bryceson, AD. Schistosomiasis in expatriates returning to Britain from the tropics: a controlled study. *Lancet*, 1986, 1(8472), 86-88.

[9] Lucey, DR; Maguire, JH. Schistosomiasis. *Infect Dis Clin North Am*, 1993, 7, 635-653.

[10] Shimazu, C; Pien, FD; Parnell, D. Bronchoscopic diagnosis of Schistosoma japonicum in a patient with hemoptysis. *Respir Med*, 1991, 85, 331-332.

[11] Schaberg, T; Rahn, W; Racz, P; Lode, H. Pulmonary schistosomiasis resembling acute pulmonary tuberculosis. *Eur Respir J*, 1991, 4, 1023-1026.

[12] Shebel, HM; Elsayes, KM; Abou, HM; Elguindy, YM; El-Diasty, TA. Genitourinary schistosomiasis: life cycle and radiologic-pathologic findings. *Radiolographics*, 2012, 32(4), 1031-1046.

[13] Baik, SK; Kim, JW; Kim, HS; Kwon, SO; Kim, YJ; Park, JW; Kim, SH; Chang, SJ; Lee, DK; Han, KH; Um, SH; Lee, SS. Recent variceal bleeding: Doppler US hepatic vein waveform in assessment of severity of portal hypertension and vasoactive drug response. *Radiology*, 2006, 240(2), 574-80.

[14] Coura, JR; Conceição, MJ. Specific schistosomiasis treatment as a strategy for disease control. *Mem. Inst. Oswaldo Cruz*, 2010, 105, 598-603.

[15] Meyer, T; Sekljic, H; Fuchs, S; Bothe, H; Schollmeyer, D; Mikulka, C. Taste, A New Incentive to Switch to (R)-Praziquantel in Schistosomiasis Treatment. (2009) *PLoS Negl Trop Dis*, 3(1), e357.

[16] Doenhoff, MJ; Jagan, P; Cioli, D; Southgate, V; Pica-Mattoccia, L; Botros, S; Coles, G; Tchuem Tchuente, LA; Mbaye, A; Engels, D. Praziquantel: its use in control of schistosomiasis in sub-Saharan Africa and current research needs. *Parasitology*, 2009, 136, 1825–1835.

[17] Jeziorski, MC; Greenberg, RM. Voltage-gated calcium channel subunits from platyhelminths: Potential role in praziquantel action. *Int J Parasitol*, 2006, 31, 625–632.

[18] Harnett, W; Kusel, JR. Increased exposure of parasite antigens at the surface of adult male *Schistosoma mansoni* exposed to praziquantel in vitro. *Parasitology*, 1986, 93, 401-405.

[19] Angelucci, F; Basso, A; Bellelli, A; Brunori, M; Pica Mattoccia, L; Valle, C. The anti-schistosomal drug praziquantel is an adenosine antagonist. *Parasitology*, 2007, 134, 1215-1221.

[20] Masimirembwa, CM; Hasler, JA. Characterisation of praziquantel metabolism by rat liver microsomes using cytochrome P450 inhibitors. *Biochem Pharmacol*, 1994, 48(9),1779-1783.

[21] Lima, RM; Ferreira, MAD; Carvalho, TM; Fernandes, BJD; Takayanagui, OM; Garcia, HH; Coelho, EB; Lanchote, VL. Albendazole-praziquantel interaction in healthy volunteers: kinetic disposition, metabolism and enantioselectivity. B*r J Clin Pharmacol.*, 2010, 71(4), 528–535.

[22] Perez del Villar, L; Burguillo, FJ; Lopez-Aban, J; Muro, A. Systematic Review and Meta-Analysis of Artemisinin Based Therapies for the Treatment and Prevention of Schistosomiasis. *PLoS ONE*, 2012, 7(9), e45867.

[23] Olliaro, PL; Vaillant, MT; Belizario, VJ; Lwambo, NJ; Ouldabdallahi, M; Pieri, OS; Amarillo, ML; Kaatano, GM; Diaw, M; Domingues, AC; Favre, TC; Lapujade, O; Alves, F; Chitsulo, L. A Multicentre Randomized Controlled Trial of the Efficacy and Safety of Single-Dose Praziquantel at 40 mg/kg vs. 60 mg/kg for Treating Intestinal Schistosomiasis in the Philippines, Mauritania, Tanzania and Brazil. *PLoS Negl Trop*, Dis 2011, 5(6), e1165.

[24] Ferrari, MLA; Coelho, PMZ; Antunes, CMF; Tavares, CAP; da Cunha, AS. Efficacy of oxamniquine and praziquantel in the treatment of Schistosoma mansoni infection: a controlled trial. *Bulletin of the World Health Organization*, 2003, 81, 190-196.
[25] Barnhill, AF; Novozhilova, E; Day, AT; Carlon, AS. Schistosoma-associated Salmonella resist antibiotic via specific fimbrial attachment to the flatworm. *Parasite and Vectors*, 2011, 123(4), 2-8.
[26] Adam, I; Elwasila, el T; Homeida, M. Is praziquantel therapy safe during pregnancy? *Trans R Soc Trop Med Hyg*, 2004, 98, 540-543.
[27] Adam, I; Elwasila, E; Homeida, M. Praziquantel for the treatment of schistosomiasis mansoni during pregnancy. *Ann Trop Med Parasitol*, 2005, 99, 37-40.
[28] Savioli, L; Crompton, DW; Neira, M. Use of anthelminthic drugs during pregnancy. *Am J Obstet Gynecol*, 2003, 188, 5-6.
[29] WHO Preventive Chemotherapy in Human Helminthiasis. (2006). WHO, Geneva.

In: Schistosomiasis
Editor: Adriana Erica Miele
ISBN: 978-1-63117-186-4

Chapter 3

Epidemiology, Chemotherapy and New Therapeutic Approaches of Schistosomiasis

Rosimeire Nunes de Oliveira**, Vera Lúcia Garcia Rehder, Tarsila Ferraz Frezza, Veronica de Lourdes Sierpe Jeraldo, Cláudia Moura de Melo and Silmara Marques Allegretti
State University of Campinas-Unicamp, Campinas, SP, Brazil,
Technological Research Institute,
Laboratory of Infectious and Parasitic Diseases, Aracaju, SE, Brazil

Abstract

Schistosomiasis, a debilitating parasitic disease caused by trematodes of the genus *Schistosoma*, is a major parasitic infection in the group of neglected tropical helminth infections, requiring more studies and specific policies for its control. This parasitosis has already been considered the most prevalent endemic among the poor rural population, especially in the northeastern states of Brazil, being, therefore, classified as "rural endemic". Even today the global strategy to control this disease

*Corresponding author: Laboratório de Helmintologia, Dep.to Biologia Animal, Instituto de Biologia, Unicamp, SP, Monteiro Lobato, 255, Bloco J, CEP 13083-862, Campinas SP, Brazil. eMail: rosy_biologa@yahoo.com.br.

is based on chemotherapy, in which praziquantel (PZQ) is the first-rate drug. Currently, the concern with tolerance and possible resistance to the treatment with PZQ, coupled with the availability of a single drug to treat schistosomiasis, has led many researchers either to improve the existing drug or to study and provide new compounds that act against this parasitosis. In this respect, the medicinal plants are shown as promising. Considering the high cost and complexity for the development of a synthetic drug, in recent years the WHO has encouraged research on medicinal plants, considering that traditional knowledge of healing action may lead to the development of new pharmaceutical products. This could happen when their constituents are not only directly used as therapeutic agents, but also as raw materials for the synthesis of pharmacologically active compounds, especially in fighting diseases that afflict the population from developing countries. The process of discovery and development of drugs is complex, lengthy and costly and is directly linked to scientific and technological innovations. Due to this information, in recent years, a new approach has been adopted in parallel to experimental investigations: *in silico* analysis. The *in silico* method helps in making decisions, predictions, hypotheses and ultimately, provides discoveries or advances in medicine and therapy. In addition to this one, a new approach called "*Drug Repurposing*" or "*Drug Repositioning*" has attracted substantial interest for some pharmaceutical industries. This approach consists in the reuse of validated drugs commonly used to treat specific diseases in order to identify new therapeutic indications to treat other diseases, thereby enhancing the industrial production and leading to new drugs for the treatment of the neglected diseases. This chapter will address, therefore, epidemiological aspects of schistosomiasis as well as a review of control strategies and chemotherapy. Finally, we shall discuss new technologies for the chemotherapy of schistosomiasis.

Keywords: Rural disease, field control strategies, *in silico* drug discovery, drug repositioning

Introduction

Schistosomiasis, a debilitating parasitic disease caused by trematodes of the genus *Schistosoma*, is a major parasitic infection in the group of neglected tropical helminth infections requiring more studies and specific policies for its control (Gryseels et al., 2006). According to the World Health Organization (WHO), approximately 243 million people were infected by this parasite in 2011 and probably 28 million received treatment, what represents only 11% of people infected worldwide (WHO, 2013). Furthermore, it is believed that schistosomiasis causes annually losses, between 1.7 and 4.5 million according to Disability Adjusted Life Years (DALY), in other words, the sum of potential years of life and years of productive life loss due to premature mortality from the disease. For this reason it is considered one of the most prevalent among the neglected parasitic diseases especially in developing countries (Parise & Silveira Filho, 2001; Utzinger & Keiser, 2004; WHO, 2004).

Despite ongoing attempts to control this infection, the guidelines of most of the helminthiasis control programs advocate mass treatment without prior diagnosis using chemical compounds listed in WHO (WHO, 2009). In areas where schistosomiasis is endemic, treatment is based on the use of praziquantel (PZQ), being it well tolerated by patients and providing therapeutic efficacy against all species of *Schistosoma* (Cioli & Pica Mattoccia, 2003; Doenhoff et al., 2008). However, dependence on only one drug is a concern, since cases of lower sensitivity to PZQ of some strains of *Schistosoma* have been reported. In addition, PZQ has some limitations such as low therapeutic efficacy on the young forms of the parasite (Doenhoff et al., 2008; Fallon et al., 1995; Gryseels et al., 2001).

Due to the high prevalence and wide epidemiological distribution of intestinal schistosomiasis, caused by *Schistosoma mansoni*, and the limitation of effective, safe and affordable drugs, it makes necessary the study of new therapeutic alternatives representing another option to the existing drug or that may be jointly used with the aim of targeting the immature stages of the parasite too. However, the pharmaceutical companies argue that research and drug development (R&D) are expensive and risky procedures to invest in neglected diseases, which predominantly affect developing countries and consequently bring a low financial return. Furthermore, only 5% of the selected drugs that undergo preclinical trials get approval for clinical use (Kola et al., 2004). Thus, it is essential an alliance between government, universities and pharmaceutical industries for the creation and maintenance of programs for R&D, focused on the study of new therapies for the control and treatment of this parasitosis (Guido & Oliva, 2009).

Epidemiology of Schistosomiasis

There are six species of *Schistosoma* that parasitize humans: *S. haematobium*, *S. japonicum*, *S. intercalatum*, *S. mekongi*, *S. malayensis* and *S.*

mansoni. However, most of the cases are ascribed to the infection by *S. haematobium* and *S. mansoni* that are antroponotic species and therefore eradicable (Gryseels, 2012). The disease is spread in 78 countries and territories.

In sub-Saharan Africa, human schistosomiasis is the second leading cause of morbidity, loosing out to malaria. The Republic of Tanzania and Nigeria have recorded approximately 93% of all the worldwide reported cases and 200, 000 deaths per year caused primarily by *S. mansoni* and S. *haematobium* (Hotez et al., 2012; Mazigo et al., 2012; Meltzer & Schwartz, 2013). It is therefore considered an endemic disease associated with socio-economic problems ravaging developing countries, where poverty and lack of sanitary infrastructure perpetuate and expand areas at risk of infection, since urbanization, precariously made over sanitation/environment and housing, allows the spreading of schistosomiasis outbreaks (Engels et al., 2002; Magalhães et al., 2011; Palmeira et al., 2010). The infection can also be favoured due to the geographic location, cultural and labor activities undertaken by the populations (Appleton & Madsen, 2012; Chitsulo et al., 2000; Meltzer & Schwartz, 2013; Tukahebwa et al., 2013).

Schistosomiasis mansoni is an endemic disease that has accompanied man since ancient times, proven by the finding of calcified eggs of *S. mansoni* in Egyptian mummies (Parise - Filho & Silveira 2001; Ziskind, 2009). Currently, this disease is endemic in 53 countries in Africa, the Middle East, the Caribbean and South America (Coura & Amaral, 2004; Murray, 2007; WHO, 2010).

In endemic areas of Africa, schistosomiasis can be found in individuals of different age groups, although children under the age of 15 have the highest rates of prevalence and intensity of infection. However, prevalence rates follow patterns related to the behaviour of individuals. In addition, the immune response may contribute to differences in the intensity of infection in different population groups (Mazigo et al., 2013). Thus, co-infections of HIV and *S. mansoni* are common in sub-Saharan Africa. Several studies have suggested possible interactions between the two infections that may affect important parameters of HIV infection, such as $CD4^+$ lymphocytes and viral loads, showing strong epidemiological evidence that the treatment of schistosomiasis would reduce the establishment of HIV virus and subsequent development of AIDS. Thereby, it is important to integrate the control programs of these two infections in that region (Gryseels et al., 2006; Mazigo et al., 2013; Secor, 2006; WHO, 2006).

The prevalence of schistosomiasis in the Americas has greatly suffered a reducing impact as a result of control campaigns that have been developed in different countries. Therefore, some Caribbean islands, Venezuela and Puerto Rico, at different scales, have managed to decrease the prevalence rates up to the elimination of the infection (Engels et al., 2002; Hyllier, 2005; Noya et al., 2006). In Venezuela, the low prevalence rates lead to a new situation, in which the infected individuals have low parasitic loads (<100 eggs/g of faeces) and bland morbidities, which translates into difficulties of detecting these clinical cases (Noya et al. 2004).

Regarding Brazil, it is believed that the introduction of schistosomiasis occurred after the arrival of African populations in the sixteenth century in the Northeast coastline. The infection was mainly expanded by large watersheds (Morgan et al., 2001; Silveira, 1989). Epidemiological studies were initiated in Brazil in the 1940s. In the '50s field researches were already carried out in communities through innovative methodologies for that time not focusing studies in patients in hospital settings. These first researches brought important contributions on vectors knowledge, transmission dynamics, epidemiology and control strategies of schistosomiasis (Coimbra Jr., 1997).

Currently, in Brazil there are approximately 25 million people living in endemic areas and probably 4.6 million infected individuals (WHO, 2010; Scholte et al., 2012; Meltzer & Schwartz, 2013). According to the Brazilian Ministry of Health, the epidemiological situation of schistosomiasis is expressed by 50% reduction in mortality and 90% in the rate of hospitalization in the period of 1990-2009. The national parasitological survey in 10, 783, 144 individuals evaluated between 2005 and 2010, revealed a quantity of 647, 861 patients with this infection (Brazil, 2010). In South America, Brazil has the most reported cases (Barakat et al., 2000). Schistosomiasis occurs in 18 states including the Federal District and is most prevalent in the Northeast region, the state of Minas Gerias, Southeast and Midwest regions (Brazil, 2009).

These endemic areas have poor hygiene and inappropriate health resources what is usually associated to poverty and low economic development (Coura-Filho, 1997). In fact, the difficulty to access health services, migration and poor water and sewage treatments are the main factors for the transmission of this parasite in these endemic areas, located in rural and urban communities (Figures 1 and 2). (Silva & Domingues, 2011; Freitas et al., 2010; Nunes et al., 2005; Souza et al., 2011).

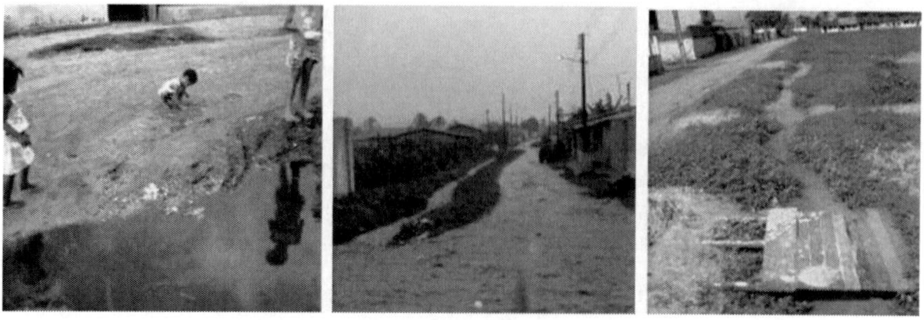

Figure 1. Precarious sanitation in urban outskirts in northeastern Brazil.

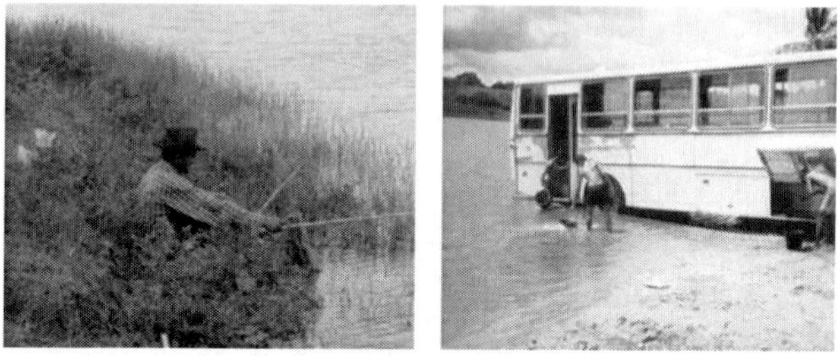

Figure 2. Standard contact with water in the rural area of northeastern Brazil: fishing activities (left panel), car wash (right panel).

In the northeastern states of Brazil, schistosomiasis has already been considered the most prevalent endemic among the poor rural population, being, therefore, classified as a "rural endemic". In 2011, over half of the cases were reported in that region with approximately 37, 000 diagnosed cases followed by 66% of deaths (Brasil, 2013).

Recent studies reveal that the epidemiological profile of the disease has undergone significant changes since it is currently transmitted in the outskirts of many cities and even in large urban centers (Massara et al., 2012; Silva & Domingues, 2011). In this region the disease has reached hyperendemic levels in all States especially in Pernambuco, Bahia, Sergipe and Alagoas. In these latter states, the epidemiological situation hasn't undergone major changes over the years despite the efforts of governmental control programs (Figure 3). Moreover, the situation is particularly worrying in the state of Alagoas where more than 12, 000 cases of the disease were diagnosed in 2011 (Brasil, 2012).

The pattern of contact with water contaminated by cercariae of the parasite occurs due to various reasons that are associated with socio-economic and cultural characteristics of the populations in endemic areas (Sarvel et al., 2011). According to sex differences, the prevalence rates of schistosomiasis in men can be attributed to behavioral aspects of male activities like sports/leisure in permanent or temporary basins (rivers and ditches), such as fishing and swimming, in addition to work activities, such as cutting grass and sand extraction, determining a higher exposure of this genre (Tukahebwa et al., 2013). In rural or transitional rural/urban environment, women use rivers for washing clothes, dishes and for bathing/hygiene, exposing themselves to infection in the same way as men (Melo et al., 2011).

On top of that, transmission through irrigated areas has been observed in Brazil. Here, for example, adult men perform work activities and children enjoy the impounding of water, exposing themselves to the parasite in places with high levels of fecal contamination (Figure 2) (Barbosa et al., 2012). In irrigated areas for rice cultivation, the prevalence in local communities can overcome 40%, but these irrigated areas are not always sources of risk. Moreover, the prevalence rates of infection in areas of mechanized work are unchanged, showing that the risk is related to the worker exposure to infected water (Barboza et al., 2012; Martins & Barreto, 2003).

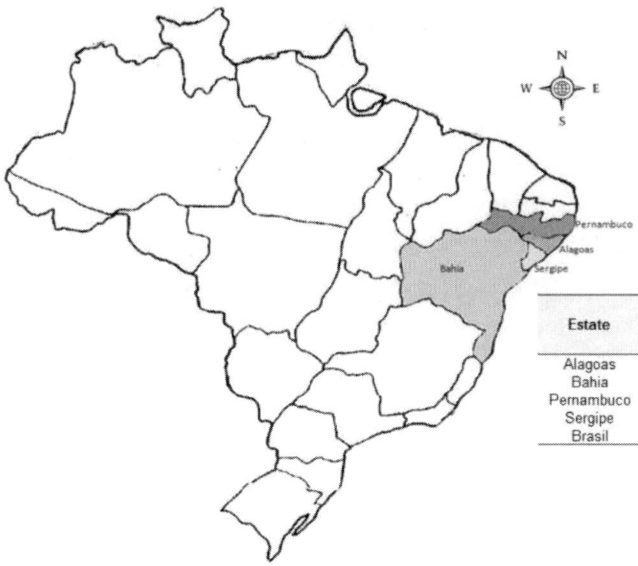

Estate	Prevalence	
	1980/1989	1990/2002
Alagoas	16,7	19,8
Bahia	10,9	9,7
Pernambuco	14,7	14,6
Sergipe	16,3	17,7
Brasil	12,5	9,2

Figure 3. Prevalence of Schistosomiasis in four Brazilian states, according to the Schistosomiasis Control Program (PCE) in the periods 1980-89 and 1990-2002. Source: Coura & Amaral, 2004.

Despite the work of prevention and control that has been developed by the Schistosomiasis Control Program (PCE) in Brazil, new foci of transmission arise because of migration of individuals from endemic areas to new areas traditionally free of infection. This situation often leads to the appearance of acute clinical cases (Lambertucci et al., 2013).

The epidemiological studies have shown a displacement of the risk areas for schistosomiasis infection (and its infection rates) related to the population density of *Biomphalaria* spp. (Gomes et al., 2012), showing the dynamics of the distribution, which certainly demands continuous evaluation and monitoring actions in situ.

Schistosomiasis mansoni also presents epidemiological relevance in developed countries where the flow of migrants and travelers from endemic regions become part of the population profile, often with asymptomatic infections that not necessarily progress to severe cases (Hatz, 2005; Schwartz, 2005).

On the other hand, in countries where the schistosomiasis control programs are being successful, such as Egypt and some Latin American countries, a new outlook is presented. In these countries, prevalence rates are underestimated by the drastic reduction of the prevalence and intensity of infections, creating a new problem concerning the loss of sensitivity of the diagnostic tools traditionally used (Enk et al., 2012).

Schistosomiasis Mansoni: Actual Chemotherapy and New Therapeutic Approaches

Chemotherapy and Chemoprophylaxis

The modern chemotherapy against schistosomiasis began with Christopherson in 1918 who reported the successful treatment of the disease in the urine (caused by *S. haematobium*), using tartar emetic antimony (Parise & Silveira Filho, 2001). Since then, several schistosomicidal compounds were studied and many were discarded due to the high toxicity and poor patient tolerance.

Later, the use of praziquantel (PZQ), started in the late 1970s, was essential to control schistosomiasis morbidity and mortality. Even today the global strategy to control this disease is based on chemotherapy in which PZQ is the first-rate drug. Its extensive use has raised concern about the development of tolerant *Schistosoma* spp. resistant to treatment (Fallon & Doenhoff, 1994).

The development of resistance to PZQ is not a consensus among the authors. According to Liu et al. (2011), there is no compelling clinical evidence of this process, indicating that the drug is still effective for *S. haematobium*, *S. mansoni* and *S. japonicum*. However, there is an agreement that tolerance in some regions is real, such as in Africa where it has been necessary to increase the dose and duration of the treatment.

It is also known that resistance can be experimentally induced in laboratory where the parasites exposed to sub-lethal concentrations for several generations produce worms less sensitive to drugs (Ismail et al., 1996; 1999; Fallon et al., 1995). The reduction of clinical cure and treatment failure of the schistosomiasis using PZQ has been reported in Egypt and Senegal (Stelma et al., 1995; Gryseels, 1994, Ismail et al., 1996; 1999), even though there is insufficient evidence that could assert and explain drug resistance in these regions (Fallon et al., 1995). According to Doenhoff et al. (2008), there is a growing number of cases of failure to the treatment of schistosomiasis with PZQ, acquired by travelers or military personnel who have been in endemic areas. These data show that, even though there isn't enough clinical evidence to prove the existence of *Schistosoma* resistance, it is prudent to take precautions to avoid it, since the existence of drug tolerance is a consonance among the authors and the "key" of the resistance process is the percentage of the survival of worms to chemotherapy that will contribute to the strength of the next generation (Ismail et al., 1999; Liang et al., 2001).

Currently, the concern with tolerance and possible resistance to the treatment with PZQ, coupled with the availability of one single drug to treat schistosomiasis, has led many researchers to improve the existing drug or to study and provide new compounds that act against this parasitosis.

One of the disadvantages of PZQ is that, although it is rapidly absorbed by the body when orally administered (about 15 minutes with peaks between 1 to 2 hours), it also rapidly disappears from circulation (within 1 to 3 hours after its ingestion), being almost completely eliminated (*via* feces and urine) in approximately 24 hours (Leopold et al., 1978; Valencia et al., 1994). Therefore, in an attempt to improve the bioavailability of the drug, increase the healing rates and reduce tolerance problems, studies were conducted on PZQ encapsulation in liposomes, i.e., microscopic vesicles containing one or more concentric spheres of lipid layers separated by an aqueous compartment (Frezza et al., 2013; Mourão et al., 2005).

Mourao et al. (2005) tested the liposomal-PZQ system *in vitro* (lip-PZQ) and proved most schistosomicide action for *S. mansoni* in relation to the free PZQ. The same authors explain that once encapsulated, drugs poorly soluble in aqueous environment, such as PZQ, display an increase of the drug availability. Frezza et al. (2013) tested the same system *in vivo* and proved the schistosomicidal action with respect to adults of *S. mansoni*, anti-oviposition and anti-granuloma formation action, when lip-PZQ is administered orally in a single dose on day 45 post infection, possibly indicating that the lip-PZQ target might be the liver and also that it could be better absorbed by the tegument of the worms, which has phospholipid affinity.

Currently, the goal of discovering new compounds that act against schistosomiasis is made through screening with isolated compounds, essential oils and organic extracts, especially extracted from plant species. The use of herbal remedies can be an alternative for the treatment of many infectious diseases (Allegretti et al., 2012; Moraes, 2012; Newman & Cragg, 2012; Kayser et al., 2003). Considering the high cost and complexity to the development of a synthetic drug, in recent years the WHO (2002) has encouraged research on medicinal plants especially in fighting diseases that afflict the population from developing countries. This is based on the consideration that traditional knowledge of healing action may lead to the development of new pharmaceutical products, when their constituents are not only directly used as therapeutic agents, but also as raw materials for the synthesis of pharmacologically active compounds. According to Lapa et al. (2007), the primary objective of preparing herbal medicines is not to replace the drugs already approved and launched in the market, but increase the therapeutic options offering similar safe drugs amplifying the action spectra. It is estimated that 25% out of $8 billion of the revenues of the pharmaceutical companies, in 1996, is due to drugs derived from different plant species (Lopez, 2006; WHO, 2006). Thus, steroidal alkaloids of fruits of *Solanum lycocarpum*, epi-isopiloturine, imidazole alkaloid isolated from the leaves of *Pilocarpus microphyllus*, the pirplatine isolated from *Piper tuberculatum*, phloroglucinol compounds from rhizomes of *Dryopteris* spp., carvacryl acetate derived from existing carvacrol in the essential oil of various species of plants, essential oils of *Baccharis trimera* (Less) and *Piper cubeba*, extracts of *Cordia verbenacea* and *Phyllanthus amarus* were objects of assays *in vitro* and *in vivo* demonstrating promising anti-schistosomiasis results (Allegretti et al., 2012; de Oliveira et al., 2012; Ferreira et al., 2011; Koné et al., 2012; Magalhães et al., 2010; Magalhães et al., 2012; Miranda et al., 2012; Moraes et al., 2011;

Moraes et al., 2013; Mostafa et al., 2011; Oliveira et al., 2013; Veras et al., 2012).

Knowing that PZQ has efficacy to treat schistosomiasis when administered between the fifth and sixth week of infection, presenting gaps between the first and fifth, it is evident that the drug shows little activity for young forms (schistosomula) of *S. mansoni* and does not eliminate the chances of reinfection (Gonnert & Andrews, 1977; Sabah et al., 1986; Webbe, 1977; Xiao et al., 1985). The moderate activity of PZQ against schistosomula indicates a low activity in the spectrum of action of this drug, and the required administration of a second dose after a short period of time to eliminate all the parasites (Doenhoff et al., 2008), therefore, compounds that act in this early stage arestrictly required. In this context, chemoprophylaxis in schistosomiasis can be defined as the prevention using compounds that act on the invasion and penetration of cercariae in the skin or in the development of juvenile worms into adults in order to prevent morbidity attributed to eggs ponded by adult females (Xiao et al., 2000).

In the 1980s, the use of artemisinin derivatives (extracted from *Artemisia annua* and called "ARTs"), such as artemether, artemisone, artelinic, artesunic acids among others, against *Schistosoma* spp. was evaluated for the first time by Chinese groups, who demonstrated that the administration of these compounds in different animals experimentally infected with *S. japonicum* caused a reduction in the parasitic load and especially a reduction of schistosomula (Chen et al., 1980; Le et al. 1982). In 1990, the use of ARTs as an antischistosomal drug was approved by the Chinese Ministry of Health (Xiao, 2005). It is worth mentioning that ARTs are still extensively used in malaria control (Krishna et al., 2008).

According to Lescano et al. (2004), after the discovery of the reduced parasitic load of *S. japonicum* in areas where malaria is co-endemic, remarkable progress was made in the study of the anti-*Schistosoma* action of artemesinin and its derivatives (ARTs), hence contemplating to enlarge the use to other continents. The use of ARTs in order to treat cases of malaria in parts of Africa, where there is an overlap with schistosomiasis, might have had a significant influence on the decreasing of morbidity of the endemic schistosomiasis (Cioli et al., 2003; Lescano et al., 2004; Lu et al. 2010; Xiao et al., 2000).

Subsequent studies extended the action of ARTs to different species of *Schistosoma* that parasitize humans. In 1984, it was demonstrated the effectiveness of these derivatives against the juvenile stages of infection, a period in which the treatment with PZQ failed (Lu et al., 2010; Yue et al.,

1984). Tests made in Brazil, in 1991, demonstrated a reduction in parasite burden in mice infected with *S. mansoni* and treated with artemether (AM) (Araujo et al., 1991). Later, it was determined that AM and artesunate (AS) exerted anti-schistosomules activity against different species of *Schistosoma* and may induce resistance to reinfection (Bergquist et al., 2009; Utzinger et al., 2002; Xiao & Catto, 1989, Xiao et al., 2000).

Liu et al. (2011) suggest that short and periodical clinical administration of AM and AS can enhance the preventive potential, especially when administered in concentrations of 6 mg/kg in 8 doses distributed at biweekly and weekly intervals, respectively. On the other hand, according to these authors, despite acting in preventing the morbidity, AM and AS do not seem to be very active in the eradication of schistosomiasis. Therefore they suggested that a combined use of PZQ + ARTs would be useful in endemic areas, where reinfections frequently occur. A recent preclinical study demonstrated the efficiency of AS against juveniles (7 and 21 day old) worms of the Egyptian lineage of *S. mansoni*, while protecting the host from damage caused by the parasite eggs and opening a discussion about the use of this compound in the control of schistosomiasis, in areas where malaria is not endemic (El-Beshbish et al., 2013). Many other studies have been conducted with ARTs for the prevention of schistosomiasis (Pérez del Villar et al., 2012). However, before they can be used in chemo-prevention of schistosomiasis more accurate studies on several other strains of the worm are needed (El- Beshbish et al., 2013).

The difference in susceptibility to ARTs related to the age of parasites is not completely understood, but may be explained by the higher quantity of anti reactive oxygen species (ROS) protective enzymes in adults than in schistosomula. This makes the juvenile worms more susceptible to free radicals released after the cleavage of the ARTS endoperoxide by haemine or other iron compounds in *Schistosoma*, causing higher mortality rates in juveniles than in adults, even using the same dose (Nare et al., 1990).

Hua et al. (2010) reported, however, that the AS sensitivity by *S. japonicum* has been decreasing over the past 10 years in China. Regarding toxicity, the ARTs are well tolerated when orally administered as demonstrated by clinical trials, indicating that side effects such as mild abdominal pain, dizziness, headache and diarrhea or slight fever appear in less than 1% of treated patients (Nontprasert et al., 2002; Wu et al., 1995).

In recent years, several studies have been conducted involving chemoprophylaxis to schistosomiasis using other compounds. Mefloquine (MQ), for example, a drug discovered in the early 1970s and used for prevention and treatment of malaria (Sweeney, 1981), has experimentally shown promising action (Manneck et al., 2010). Proof-of-concept trials have been made on *S. mansoni* and *S. haematobium* in children infected by these parasites in regions where malaria and schistosomiasis are co-endemic (Keiser et al., 2009).

In vitro studies conducted by Manneck et al. (2010) demonstrated that MQ has rapid action against schistosomula, killing the worms between 1 and 6 hours with sub-lethal concentrations. In contrast, the adult worms have a slow response to the addition of MQ in a culture medium in which the peak of the mortality rate was observed within 24 hours, always at sub-lethal concentrations. The electronic scanning microscopy revealed that the MQ causes extensive tissue damage in both juvenile and adult worms. *In vivo* trials conducted by the same authors showed higher percentage of worms in the liver (hepatic shift) than in mesenteric veins compared to the control group, when mice were treated with MQ 400 mg/kg in a single oral dose, between 7 and 8 weeks post infection. The mechanism of action of MQ in schistosomules is not completely elucidated, but it is suggested that this compound acts as a glycolysis inhibitor *via* the enolase, at least in stages where other targets, such as haemine degradation, are not relevant (Manneck et al., 2012).

The schistosomicidal action of 8-Hydroxyquinoline (8-HQ) derivatives, a known iron chelator with anti-oxidant properties and major constituents of a pharmaceutical compounds class, has been reported by Soliman & Hammouda (1979) and Soliman et al., (1984). Recently, the activity of new 8-HQ derivatives acting against adults and juveniles *S. mansoni*, as well as their action against granuloma, was evaluated *in vivo* by Allam et al. (2013). Oral administration of these compounds at concentrations between 200 and 1000 mg/kg administered on two consecutive days, was shown to have schistosomicidal activity to both adults and juveniles worms (administration of the compounds after 8 weeks of infection) and also to the granulomatous reaction. The same authors showed that 8-HQ derivatives induce increased levels of IgG, which may indicate the induction of a protective immunity to reinfection. The exact mechanism of schistosomicidal action of both old and new 8-HQ derivatives is not yet known, but it might be related to the inhibition of thioredoxin glutathione reductase (TGR) (Eweas et al., 2013a, 2013b; Kuntz et al., 2007) associated to Fe chelation and the induction of an effective humoral immune response against the adults of *S. mansoni* (Allam et al., 2013).

Among the compounds of natural origin, isolated from medicinal plants, piplartine, a starch isolated from *Piper tuberculatum*, had an anti-schistosomules action assessed *in vitro* by Moraes et al. (2012). Feasibility studies and cutaneous destruction assessed *via* confocal laser scanning microscopy showed that this compound acts against juvenile worms, showing a better efficacy compared to PZQ. However, most researches on the activity of the natural compounds against schistosomiasis focus on their action mainly against the adult forms of the parasite. Furthermore, most of the studies show only *in vitro* screenings and require subsequent *in vivo* studies.

In Silico Discovery of Therapeutic Targets

Significant advances in research aimed at finding new drugs for the treatment of neglected diseases came from the adoption of strategies based on the evolutionary processes of molecular recognition, in order to find potential therapeutic targets.

According to Guido & Andricopulo (2008), the process of discovery and development of drugs is complex, lengthy and costly and is directly linked to scientific and technological innovations. Due to this information, in recent years, a new approach has been adopted to complement the experimental investigations: the *in silico* analysis.

The term "*in silico*" is a method adopted in pharmacology for drug discovery through computational experiments that uses various bioinformatics software in order to capture, analyze and integrate biological data. This method is directly related to the traditional biological methods *in vitro* and *in vivo*. In addition, the *in silico* method helps in making decisions and simulations that can be used to make predictions, hypotheses and that, ultimately, might boost discoveries or advances in medicine and therapy (Ekins, 2005).

According to Verlinde et al. (2001), the planning of drugs with antiparasitic activity is based mainly on the host-parasite relationship, hence it is essential to study the biochemical pathways of the parasite in order to identify possible targets that can assist the selection and modulation of bioactive molecules.

It is known that the main obstacle for the optimization of many pre-clinical and clinical studies is the difficulty of capturing and integrating relevant information about molecules and specific targets responsible for the lethal effect of the pathogenic agents without harming its host. In this sense, it was created the open access database TDRtargets (http://tdrtargets.org/) maintained by the Special Programme for Research and Training in Tropical Diseases (TDR). This tool has been used to facilitate multiple approaches and to detect potential pharmacological targets, prioritizing the identification of specific genes and proteins, especially for the treatment of neglected diseases such as schistosomiasis, trypanosomiasis, malaria, leishmaniasis, sleeping sickness. It has also been widely used as support for further experimental studies (Crowther et al., 2010).

The successful use of the *in silico* method, including the identification of proteins, enzymes and genes as potential therapeutic targets has been described. Liu et al. (2013) conducted one *in silico*-integrated *in vitro* study, which included thirty bioactive molecules. Using molecular docking they found that 3-oxoacyl-ACP Reductase (OAR), a key enzyme involved in synthesis of fatty acids, was a potential target for the development of new drugs against pathogens. To confirm the simulations, it's *in vitro* schistosomicidal activity was investigated.

Anderson et al. (2012) evaluated the interaction of histones Small Heterodimer Partner (SHP) from *S. mansoni* with histone acetyltransferases, methyltransferases and deacetylases (HDACs) and showed that it was a potential therapeutic target raising an apoptotic phenotype further to the inhibition of HDAC. According to the authors, a deeper knowledge of histones modifications opens the way to a better understanding of genes regulation in *S. mansoni* and to the possible use of SHP as a target for the development of new drugs.

Caffrey et al. (2009) used the *in silico* method to compare the proteome of *S. mansoni* with two experimental models, used to identify potential drug targets against helminths, *Caenorhabditis elegans* and *Drosophila melanogaster*. The study showed that a set of proteins with functions in orthologous gene disruption had sequences similar to the antigens of the parasite eggs. The different expression of these latter caused disorders, changes in motility and lethal effects to different developmental stages of the parasite.

Considering the importance and necessity of developing new active ingredients for the treatment of schistosomiasis, the *in silico* method offers new strategies to identify specific therapeutic targets and arouses the interest of the pharmaceutical industry, since experimental investigations, including *in vitro* and *in vivo* screening, are expensive and require a long timeframe, especially when a given pharmacological target needs to be specific for the different stages of the life cycle of a given pathogen (Anishetty et al., 2005; Caffrey et al., 2009).

Drug Repositioning

In recent years, a new approach called "*Drug Repurposing*" or "*Drug Repositioning*" has attracted substantial interest from some pharmaceutical industries. This approach consists in the "reuse" of validated drugs commonly used to treat specific diseases in order to identify new therapeutic indications to treat other diseases, thereby enhancing the industrial production. In this sense, the first studies named "Drug Repurposing" were directed to the discovery of new drugs designed for the treatment of obesity and Parkinson's disease (Ashburn, 2004).

Traditionally, parasitic diseases have not been a major pharmaceutical interest, since these diseases affect low-income populations in developing countries, which makes it difficult to marketing medicines, even though they affect millions of people and have high morbidity and mortality rates (Eknis et al., 2011). However, the development of parasite tolerance and resistance to drugs commonly used in programs to control parasitosis drives further research to the discovery of new active principles, mainly in Academia, governmental research centers and in some biotech companies.

Despite the efforts to control schistosomiasis, this parasitic disease remains neglected especially in most African, Asian and some countries of Central and South America. A promising alternative to the dependence on only praziquantel (PZQ) consists in the reuse of existing drugs, optimizing experimental studies, directing them to different therapeutic targets and, thus, originating second-generation drugs (Angelucci et al., 2009). According to Uliana (2009) the "Drug Repurposing" opens new perspectives and can become an important tool for the discovery of new drugs as options for the treatment of the neglected diseases.

The governmental incentives for R&D of antimalarial and antischistosome drugs have intensified due concomitant infections in the developing countries of malaria, schistosoma, HIV and tuberculosis, affecting thousands of people and causing high morbidity and mortality (Kaiser et al., 2012; Lescano et al., 2004). Some studies have reported the effectiveness of "Drug Repurposing" of some active ingredients used in the treatment of other parasitic diseases with promising activity in the treatment of schistosomiasis. The first discoveries of the schistosomicidal activity of antimalarial drugs began in 1980, when it was found that the administration of artemisinin in animals experimentally infected with *S. japonicum* caused a significant reduction in parasitic intensity, when compared with infected and untreated animals from the control group (Utzinger et al., 2001). One reason for the repositioning of antimalarial drugs

(Table 1) is directly related to the similarity in feeding and metabolism of both parasites, *Plasmodium* and *Schistosoma* (Sophie et al., 2013).

Finally, "Drug Repurposing" and the discovery of new therapeutic targets may simplify the steps for the development of drugs reducing the time and the expenses of the process.

Table 1. Description of active molecules used in the treatment of other diseases with therapeutic targets for schistosomiasis

Active compound	Original use	Proposed new use	Method of discovery	References
Mefloquine	Antimalarial	Schistosomicidal	Assays *in vitro* and *in vivo* against life stages: Schistosomula, juvenile and adult worms	Manneck et al. (2011); Holtfreter et al. (2011); Ingram et al. (2012)
Primaquine	Antimalarial	Schistosomicidal	Assays *in vitro* and *in vivo* against schistosomula, juvenile and adult worms	Holtfreter et al. (2011)
Chloroquine	Antimalarial	Schistosomicidal	Inhibition of formation of Hemozoíne (Hz) in *S. mansoni*	Oliveira et al. (2004)
Artemisinins	Antimalarial	Schistosomicidal	Assays *in vitro* and *in vivo* against schistosomules, juvenile and adult worms	El-Lakkany et al.(2013)
Ozonides	Antimalarial	Schistosomicidal	Assays *in vivo* against schistosomules, juvenile and adult worms	Xiao et al. (2007); Keiser et al. (2012)
Trioxaquines	Antimalarial	Schistosomicidal	Assays *in vivo* and *in vivo* against cercariae, schistosomules and adult worms	Portela et al. (2012)
Miltefosine	Anti leishmaniasis	Schistosomicidal	Molluscicidal and Larvicidal (ovicidal, miracidicidal and cercaricidal) activityAssays *in vitro* against adult worms	Eissa et al. (2011)

Conclusion

Although several studies have been directed to control schistosomiasis, this disease continues to be a major worldwide public health problem with negative consequences in developing countries.

This situation has important sociocultural and ecological components. In endemic countries, where irrigation practices are being implemented, the appearance of new foci can be observed, enlightening the adaptability of vectors and promoting situations of extreme heterogeneity that require further studies in order to improve the understanding of the epidemiological aspects of the infection.

The human being acts as the main link in the epidemiological chain and has a key role in the new environments, where the endemic settles. Thus, the growth of cities, which allows the input of individuals from rural areas, an historical source of infection, associated with social problems, such as lack of health infrastructure, public health and education, create a new landscape and contribute to spread and perpetuate this parasitic disease.

In conclusion, concerning the treatment of helminthiasis, scientific and technological advances have lately provided important information for the discovery of new therapeutic targets and drug options, providing, consequently, opportunities and challenges in the R&D area. These advancements have aroused the interest of the pharmaceutical industry, since the new techniques, covered in this chapter, have facilitated the identification of drugs/lead compounds together with new therapeutic targets, thus contributing to a promising future in the treatment of this neglected disease.

Acknowledgements

The authors are grateful to Coordenação de Aperfeiçoamento de Pessoal de Nível Superior (CAPES, Brazil) and Conselho Nacional de Desenvolvimento Científico e Tecnológico (CNPq, Brazil) for financial support.

References

Allam, G., Eweas, A. F. & Abuelsaad, A. S. A. (2013). In vivo schistosomicidal activity of three novels 8-hydroxyquinoline derivatives against adult and immature worms of Schistosoma mansoni. *Parasitol Res*, *112*, 3137-3149.

Allegretti, S. M., de Oliveira, C. F. N., de Oliveira, R. N., Frezza, T. F. & Rehder, V. L. G. (2012). The use of Brazilian medicinal plants to combat Schistosoma mansoni. In: Rokni M. B. (ed) Schistosomiasis, In Tech, Rijeka, 27-70.

Anderson, L., Pierce, R. J. & Verjovski-Almeida, S. (2012). Schistosoma mansoni histones: From transcription to chromatin regulation, an in silico analysis. *Mol Biochem Parasitol*, *183*, 105–114.

Angelucci, F., Sayed, A. A., Williams, D. L., Boumis, G., Brunori, M., Dimastrogiovanni, D., Miele, A. E., Pauly, F. & Bellelli, A. (2009). Inhibition of Schistosoma mansoni thioredoxin-glutathione reductase by auranofIn: structural and kinetic aspects. *J Biol Chem*. *284*, 28977-28985.

Anishetty S., Pulimi M. & Pennathur, G. (2005). Potential drug targets in Mycobacterium tuberculosis through metabolic pathway analysis. *Comput Biol Chem*, *29*, 368–378.

Appleton, C. C. & Madsen, H. (2012). Human schistosomiasis in wetlands in southern Africa. *Wetlands Ecol Manag*, *20*, 253–269.

Araujo, N., Kohn, A. & Katz, N. (1991). Activity of the artemether in experimental Schistosoma mansoni. *Mem Inst Oswaldo Cruz*, *86*, 185-188.

Ashburn, T. T. & Thor, K. B. (2004). Drug repositioning: identifying and developing new uses for existing drugs. *Nat Rev Drug Discov*, *3*, 673–683.

Barakat, R., Farghaly, A., El-Masry, A. G., El-Sayed, M. K. & Hussein, M. H. (2000). The epidemiology of schistosomiasis in Egypt: patterns of Schistosoma mansoni infection and morbidity in Kafr el-sheikh. *Am J Trop Med Hyg*, *62*, S21-S27.

Barboza D. F. M. et al. (2012). Biomphalaria species distribution and its effect on human Schistosoma mansoni infection in an irrigated area used for rice cultivation in northeast Brazil. *Geospatial Health*, *6*, S103-S109.

Bergquist R., Johansen M. V. & Utzinger, J. (2009). Diagnostic dilemmas in helmintology: what tools to use and when? *Trends Parasitol*, *25*, 151-156.

BRASIL, Ministério da Saúde. (2009). Guia de vigilância epidemiológica. Brasília: Normas e Manuais Técnicos. 816.

BRASIL. Ministério da Saúde (2013). Sistema de informação de agravos de notificação/ Sistema de informação da esquistossomose. Óbitos por Esquistossomose. Brasil, Grandes Regiões e Unidades Federadas. 1990-2011. Brasília, 2013. Available at: http://portal.saude.gov.br/portal/arquivos/pdf/obitos_esquistossomose_25_03_2013.pdf

BRASIL. Ministério da Saúde. (2012). Sistema de informação de agravos de notificação/ Sistema de informação da esquistossomose. Casos confirmados de Esquistossomose. Brasil, Grandes Regiões e Unidades Federadas. 1995 a 2011. Brasília, 2012. Available at: http://portal.saude.gov.br/portal/arquivos/pdf/serie_historica_esquistossomose_07_08_2012.pdf

BRASIL. Ministério da Saúde. Secretaria de Vigilância em Saúde. (2010). Situação epidemiológica da esquistossomose no Brasil, Brasília: Editora do Ministério da Saúde.

BRASIL. Ministério da Saude. (2006). Política nacional de plantas medicinais e fitoterápicos. Secretaria de Ciência, Tecnologia e Insumos Estratégicos. Departamento de Assistência Farmacêutica e Insumos Estratégicos – Brasília.

Caffrey, C. R., et al. (2009). A Comparative Chemogenomics Strategy to Predict Potential Drug Targets in the Metazoan Pathogen, *Schistosoma mansoni*. *PLoS One*, *4*, e4413.

Chen, D. J., et al. (1980). Studies on antischistosomal activity of qinghaosu in experimental therapy. *Zhong Hui Yi Xue Zha Zhi*, *80*, 422-428.

Chitsulo, L., Engels, D., Montresor, A. & Savioli L. (2000). The global status of schistosomiasis and its control. *Acta Trop*, *77*, 41–51.

Christopheron, J. B. (1918). The successful use of antimony in bilharziosis. Administered as intravenous injections of antimonium tartaratum (tartar emetic). *Lancet*, *192*, 325-327.

Cioli, D. & Pica-Mattoccia, L. (2003). Praziquantel. *Parasitol Res*, *90*, S3-S9.

Coimbra, Jr C. E. A. (1997). Uma conversa com Frederico Simões Barbosa. *Cadernos de Saúde Pública*, *13*, 564-565.

Coura-FIilho, P. C. (1997). Distribuição da esquistossomose no espaço urbano. 2. Aproximação teórica sobre a acumulação, concentração, centralização do capital e a produção de doenças. *Cadernos de Saúde Pública*, *13*, 415-424.

Coura J. R. & Amaral, R. S. P. (2004). Epidemiological and control aspects of schistosomiasis in Brazilian endemic areas. *Mem Inst Oswaldo Cruz*, *99*, 3-19.

Crowter, G. J., et al. (2010). Identification of Attractive Drug Targets in Neglected- Disease Pathogens Using an In silico Appoach. *PLoS Negl Trop Dis*, *48*, e804.

De Oliveira, R. N., et al. (2012). Schistosoma mansoni, in vitro schistosomicidal activity of essential oil of Baccharis trimera (less) DC. *Exp Parasitol*, *132*, 135-143.

Dohenoff, M. J., Cioli, D. & Utzinger, J. (2008). Praziquantel, mechanism of action, resistance and new derivatives for schistosomiasis. *Curr Opin Infect Dis*, *21*, 659-667.

Eissa, M. H., El-Azzouni, M. Z., Amer E. I. & Baddour N. M. (2011). Miltefosine, a promising novel agent for Schistosomiasis mansoni. *Int J Parasitol*, *41*, 235-242.

Ekins, S. et al. (2005). Systems biology: applications in drug discovery. In Drug discovery Handbook (Gad, S., ed.), 123–183.

Ekins, S., Williams, A. J., Matthew, D., Krasowski, M. D. & Freundlich, J. S. (2011). In silico repositioning of approved drugs for rare and neglected diseases. *Drug Discov Today*, *16*, 298-310.

El-Beshbishi, S. N., Taman, A., El-Malky, M., Azab, M. S., El-Hawary, A. K. & El-Tantawy, D. A. (2013). In vivo effect of single oral dose of artemether against early juvenile stages of Schistosoma mansoni Egyptian strain. *Exp Parasitol.*, *135*, 240-245.

El-Lakkany, N. M. & Seif El-DIn: S. H. (2013). Haemin enhances the in vivo efficacy of artemether against juvenile and adult Schistosoma mansoni in mice. *Parasitol Res*, *112*, 2419-2420.

Engels D., Chitsulo L., Montresor, A. & Savioli, L. (2002). The global epidemiological situation of schistosomiasis and new approaches to control and research. *Acta Trop*, *82*, 139–146.

Enk, M. J., Silva, G. O. & Rodrigues, N. B. (2012). Diagnostic accuracy and applicability of a PCR system for the detection of Schistosoma mansoni DNA in human urine samples from an endemic area. *PLoS One*, *7*, e38947.

Eweas, A. F., Allam, G., Abuelsaad, A. S., Al Ghamdi, A. H. & Maghrabi, I. A. (2013b). Design, synthesis, anti-schistosomal activity and molecular docking of novel 8- hydroxyquinoline-5-sufonyl 1, 4-diazepine derivatives. *Bioorg Chem*, *46*, 17-25.

Eweas, A. F., Allam, G., Abu-Elsaad, A. S., Maghrabi, I. A. & Al-Ghamdi, A. H. (2013a). Synthesis, anti-schistosomal activity and molecular modeling of two novel 8-hydroxyquinoline derivatives. *Anti-Infect Agents.*, *11*, 31-40.

Fallon, P. G. & Dohenoff, M. J. (1994). Drug-resistant schistosomiasis: resistance to praziquantel and oxamniquine induced in Schistosoma mansoni in mice is drug specific. *Am J Trop Med Hyg*, *53*, 61-62.

Fallon, P. G., Sturrock, R. F., Niang, A. C. & Doenhoff, M. J. (1995). Short report: diminished susceptibility to praziquantel in a Senegal isolate of Schistosoma mansoni. *Am J Trop Med Hyg.*, *53*, 61-62.

Ferreira, J. F., Peaden, P. & Keiser, J. (2011). In vitro trematocidal effects of crude alcoholic extracts of Artemisia annua, A. absinthium, Asimina triloba, and Fumaria officinalis: trematocidal plantalcoholic extracts. *Parasitol Res*, *109*, 1585-1592.

Freitas, A. R. R., Ooliveira, A. C. P. & Jachinto Silva, L. J. (2010). Schistosomal myeloradiculopathy in a low-prevalence area: 27 cases (14 autochthonous) in Campinas, São Paulo, Brazil. *Mem Inst Adolfo Lutz*, *105*, 398-408.

Frezza, T. F., et al. (2013). Liposomal-praziquantel: efficacy against Schistosoma mansoni in a preclinical assay. *Acta Trop*, *128*, 70-75.

Gomes, E. C. S., Leal-Neto, O. B., Albuquerque J., Silva, H. P. & Barbosa, C. S. (2012). Schistosomiasis transmission and environmental change: a spatio-temporal analysis in Porto de Galinhas, Pernambuco – Brazil. *Int J Health Geograph*, *11*, 51.

Gonnert, R. & Andrews, P. (1977). Praziquantel, a new broad-spectrum antischistosomal agent. *Parasitol Res*, *52*, 129-150.

Gryseels, B. Schistosomiasis. (2012). *Infect Dis Clin North Am*, *26*, 383–397.

Gryseels, B., et al. (1994). Epidemiology, immunology and chemotherapy of Schistosoma mansoni infections in a recently exposed community in Senegal. *Trop Geogr Med*, *46*, 209–219.

Gryseels, B., Polman, K., Clerinx, J. & Kestens, L. (2006). Human schistosomiasis. *Lancet*, *368*, 1106–1118.

Gryseels, B. et al. (2001). Are poor responses to praziquantel for the treatment of Schistosoma mansoni infections in Senegal due to resistance? An overview of the evidence. *Trop Med Intern Health*, *6*, 864-873.

Guido, R. V. C. & Andricopoulo, A. D. (2008). Modelagem molecular de fármacos. *Revista Procedimentos Químicos*, *2*, 24-26.

Guido, R. V. C. & Oliva, G. (2009). Structure-based drug discovery for tropical diseases. *Curr. Top Med Chem*, *9*, 824-843.

Hatz, C. (2005). Schistosomiasis: an underestimated problem in industrialised countries? *J Travel Med*, *12*, 1–2.

Hillyer, G. V. (2005). The rise and fall of Bilharzia in Puerto Rico: Its centennial 1904-2004. *P R Health Sci J*, *24*, 225-235.

Holtfreter, M. C., Loebermann, M., Klammt, S., Sombetzki, M., Bodammer, P., Riebold, D., Kinzelbach, R. & Reisinger, E. C. (2001). Schistosoma mansoni, schistosomicidal effect of mefloquine and primaquine in vitro. *Exp Parasitol.*, *127*, 270-276.

Hotez, P. J., Asojo, O. A. & Adesina, A. M. (2012). Nigeria: "Ground Zero" for the High Prevalence Neglected Tropical Diseases. *PLoS Negl Trop Dis*, *6*, e1600.

Hua, H. Y., Liang, Y. S., Zhang, Y., Wei, J.F. & Guo, H. X. (2010). The sensitivity of artesunate against Schistosoma japonicum decreased after 10 years of use in China. *Parasitol Res*, *107*, 873-878.

Ingram, K., Ellis, W. & Keiser, J. (2012). Antischistosomal activities of mefloquine- related arylmethanols. *Antimicrob Agents Chemother*, *56*, 3207-3215.

Ismail, M., et al. (1999). Resistance to praziquantel: direct evidence from Schistosoma mansoni isolated from egyptian villagers. *Am J Trop Med Hyg*, *60*, 932-935.

Ismail, M., Metwally, A., Farghaly, A., Bruce, J., Tao, L. F. & Bennett, J. L. (1996). Characterization of isolates of Schistosoma mansoni from Egyptian villagers that tolerate high doses of praziquantel. *Am J Trop Med Hyg*, *55*, 214-218.

Keiser, J., Chollet, J., Xiao, S. H., Mei, J. Y., Jiao, P. Y., Utzinger, J. & Tanner, M. (2009). Mefloquine – an antimonialcohol with promising antischistosomal properties in mice. *PloS Negl Trop Dis. 3*, e350.

Keiser, J., Ingram, K., Vargas, M., Chollet, J., Wang, X., Dong, Y. & Vennerstrom, J. L. (2012). In vivo activity of aryl ozonides against Schistosoma species. *Antimicrob Agents Chemother*. *56*, 1090-1092.

Keiser, J. & Utzinger, J. (2012). Antimalarials in the Treatment of Schistosomiasis. *Curr Pharm Des*, *18*, 3531-3538.

Keiser, O., Kiderlan, A. F. & Croft, S. L. (2003). Natural products as antiparasitic drugs. *Parasitol Res*, *90*, S55–S62.

Kola, I. & Landis, J. (2004). Can the pharmaceutical industry reduce attrition rates? *Nat Rev Drug Discov*, *3*, 711–716.

Koné, W.M., Vargas, M. & Keiser, J. (2012). Anthelminthic activity of medicinal plants used in Côte d'Ivoire for treating parasitic diseases. *Parasitol Res*, *110*, 2351-2362.

Krishna, S., Bustamante, L., Haynes, R. K. & Staines, H. M. (2008). Artemisinins: their growing importance in medicine. *Trends Pharmacol Sci*, *29*, 520-527.

Kuntz, A. N., Davioud-Charvet, E., Sayed, A. A., Califf, L. L., Dessolin, J., Arnér, E. S. & Williams, D. L. (2007). Thioredoxin glutathione reductase from Schistosoma mansoni: an essential parasite enzyme and a key drug target. *PloS Med*, *4*, e206.

Lambertucci, J. R., et al. (2013). An Outbreak of Acute Schistosoma mansoni Schistosomiasis in a Nonendemic Area of Brazil: A Report on 50 Cases, Including 5 With Severe Clinical Manifestations. *Clin Infect Dis*, *57*, e 01-e06.

Lapa, J. A., Succar, C., Lena-Landman, M. T. R., Godinho, R. O. & Nogueira, M.T.C. (2007). Farmacologia e Toxocologia de Produtos Naturais. In: *Farmacognosia da Planta ao Medicamento*. 6ª edição, editora UFRGS, p.247.

Le, W. J., You, J. Q., Yang, Y. Q., Mei, J. Y., Guo, H. F., Yang, H. Z. & Zhang, Z. W. (1982). Studies on the efficacy of artemether in experimental schistosomiasis. *Acta Phama Sinica*, *17*, 187-193.

Leopold G., Ungethum, W., Groll, E., Diekman, H. W., Nowak, H. & Wegner, D. H. (1978). Clinical pharmacology in normal volunteers of praziquantel, a new drug against schistosomes and cestodes. An example of a complex study covering both tolerance and pharmacocinetics. *Eur J Clin Pharmacol*, *14*, 281-291.

Lescano, S. Z., Chieffi P. P., Canhassi, R. R., Boulos, M. & Neto, V. A. (2004). Antischistosomal activity of artemether in experimental Schistosomiasis mansoni. *Revista de Saúde Pública*, *31*, 71-75.

Liang, Y. S., Coles, G., Dohenoff, M. J. & Vaughan, R. S. (2001). In vitro responses of praziquantel-resistant and susceptible Schistosoma mansoni to praziquantel. *Int J Parasitol*, *31*, 1227-1235.

Liu, J., et al. (2013). 3-Oxoacyl-ACP Reductase from Schistosoma japonicum, Integrated In Silico -In Vitro Strategy for Discovering Antischistosomal Lead Compounds. *PLoS One*, *8*, e64984.

Liu, R., Dong, H. F., Guo, Y., Zhao, Q. P. & Jiang, M. S. (2011). Efficacy of praziquantel and artemisinin derivatives for the treatment and prevention of human schistosomiasis: a systematic review and meta-analysis. *Parasit Vectors*, *4*, 201.

Lopez, C. A. A. (2006). Considerações gerais sobre plantas medicinais. *Ambiente*: *Gestão e Desenvolvimento*., *1*, 19-27.

Lu, G., et al. (2010). Effect of artmether, hemin and Fe3+ on recombinant lactate dehydrigenase from Schistosoma japonicum. *Asian Pac J Trop Med*, *3*, 930-933.

Magalhães, L. G., et al. (2012). In vitro efficacy of the essential oil of Piper cubeba L. (Piperaceae) against Schistosoma mansoni. *Parasitol Res, 110,* 1747-1754.

Magalhães, L. G., Kapadia, G. J., da Silva Tonuci, L. R., Caixeta, S. C., Parreira, N. A., Rodrigues, V. & Da Silva Filho, A. A. (2010). In vitro schistosomicidal effects of some phloroglucinol derivatives from Dryopteris species against Schistosoma mansoni adult worms. *Parasitol Res, 106,* 395-401.

Manneck, T., Braissant, O., Ellis, W. & Keiser, J. (2011). Schistosoma mansoni: Antischistosomal activity of the four optical isomers and the two racemates of mefloquine on schistosomula and adult worms in vitro and in vivo. *Exp Parasitol, 127,* 260–269.

Manneck, T., Haggenmueller, Y. & Keiser, J. (2010). Morphological effects and tegumental alterations induced by mefloquine on schistosomula and adult flukes of Schistosoma mansoni. *Parasitology, 137,* 85-98.

Manneck, T., Keiser, J. & Mueller, J. (2012). Mefloquine interferes with glycolysis in schistosomula of Schistosoma mansoni via enolase. *Parasitology, 139,* 497-505.

Martins, D. F. & Barreto, M. L. (2003). Aspectos macroepidemiológicos da esquistossomose mansônica: análise da relação da irrigação no perfil espacial da endemia no Estado da Bahia, Brasil. *Cadernos de Saúde Pública, 19,* 383-393.

Massara, C. L., Amaral, G. L., Caldeira, R. L., Drummond, S. C., Enk, M. J. & Omar Carvalho, O. S. (2008). Esquistossomose em área de ecoturismo do Estado de Minas Gerais, Brasil. *Cadernos de Saúde Pública, 24,* 1709-1712.

Mazigo, H. D., et al. (2012). Epidemiology and control of human schistosomiasis in Tanzania. *Parasit Vectors, 5,* 274-294.

Mazigo H. D., et al. (2013). Epidemiology and interactions of Human Immunodeficiency Virus – 1 and Schistosoma mansoni in sub-Saharan Africa. *Infect Dis Poverty,* **2**, 2-11.

Melo, A. G. S., Melo, C. M., Oliveira, C. C. C., Oliveira, D. S., Santos, V. B. & Jeraldo, V. L. S.(2011) Esquistossomose em área de transição rural-urbana, reflexões epidemiológicas. *Ciencia, Cuidado & Saúde, 10,* 506-513.

Meltzer, E. & Schwartz, E. (2013). Schistosomiasis: Current Epidemiology and Management in Travelers. *Curr Infect Dis Reports, 15,* 211–215.

Miranda, M. A., et al. (2012). Evaluation of the schistosomicidal activity of the steroidal alkaloids from Solanum lycocarpum fruits. *Parasitol Res, 111*, 257-262.

Moraes, J., et al. (2013). Anthelmintic activity of carvacryl acetate against Schistosoma mansoni. *Parasitol Res, 112*, 603-610.

Moraes, J., Nascimento, C., Lopes, P. O., Nakano, E., Yamaguchi, L. F., Kato, M. J. & Kawano, T. (2011). Schistosoma mansoni, in vitro schistosomicidal activity of piplartine. *Exp Parasitol. 127*, 357-364.

Moraes, J., Nascimento, C., Yamaguchi, L. F., Kato, M. J. & Nakano, E. (2012). Schistosoma mansoni: in vitro schistosomicidal activity and tegumental alterations induced by piplartine on schistosomula. *Exp Parasitol, 132*, 222-227.

Morgan, J. A. T., Dejong, R. J., Snyder, S. D., Koji, G. M. & Loker, E. S. (2001). Schistosoma mansoni and Biomphalaria: past history and future trends. *Parasitology, 123*, 211-228.

Mostafa, O. M., Eid, R. A. & Adly, M. A. (2011). Antischistosomal activity of ginger (Zingiber officinale) against Schistosoma mansoni harbored in C57 mice. *Parasitol Res, 109*, 395-403.

Mourao, S. C., Costa, P. I., Salgado, H. R. N. & Gremiao, M. P. (2005). Improvement of antischistosomal activity of praziquantel by incorporation into phosphatidylcholine-containing liposomes. *Int J Pharmaceutics, 295*, 157–162.

Murray, C. J. L., et al. (2007). Global burden of disease 2005: call for collaborators. *Lancet, 370*, 109-10.

Nare, B., Smith, J. M. & Prichard, R. K. (1990). Schistosoma mansoni: levels of antioxidants and resistance to oxidants increase during development. *Exp Parasitol, 70*, 389-397.

Newman, D. J. & Cragg, G. M. (2012). Natural products as sources of new drugs over the 30 years from 1981 to 2010. *J Natural Prod, 75*, 311– 335.

Nontprasert, A., Pukrittayakamee, S., Dondorp, A. M., Clemens, R., Looareesuwan, S. & White, N. J. (2002). Neuropathologic toxicity of artemisinin derivatives in a mouse model. *Am J Trop Med Hyg., 67*, 423-429.

Noya, B. A., Ruiz–Guevara, R., Colmenares, C., Losada, S. & Noya, O. (2006). Low transmission areas of schistosomiasis in Venezuela, consequences on the diagnosis, treatment, and control. *Mem Inst Oswaldo Cruz, 101*, 29-35.

Noya, B. A., Ruiz, R., Colmenares, C., Losada, S., Cesari, I. M., Toro, J. & Noya, O. (2004). Schistosomiasis mansoni in areas of low transmission.

Epidemiological characterization of Venezuelan foci. *Mem Inst Oswaldo Cruz*, *97*, 5-10.

Nunes, F. C., Costa, M. C. E., Filhote, M. I. F. & Sharapinn, M. (2005). The epidemiologic profile of the Schistosomiasis mansoni in the Alto da Boa Vista, neighborhood in Rio de Janeiro. *Cadernos Saúde Coletiva*, *13*, 605 – 616.

Oliveira C. N. F., De Oliveira, R. N., Frezza, T. F., Rehder, V. L. G. & Allegretti, S. M. (2013). Tegument of Schistosoma mansoni as a Therapeutic Target. In: *Parasitic Diseases - Schistosomiasis*, *1*, 151-177.

Oliveira, M. F., et al. (2004). Inhibition of heme aggregation by chloroquine reduces Schistosoma mansoni infection. *J Infec Dis*, *190*, 843-852.

Plameira, D. C. C, Carvalho, A. G., Rodrigues, K. & Couto, J. L.A. (2010). Prevalência da infecção pelo Schistosoma mansoni em dois municípios do Estado de Alagoas. *Revista Sociedade Brasileira Medicina Tropical*, *43*, 313-317.

Parise-Filho, R. & Siilveira, M. A. B. (2001). Current world schistosomiasis overview. *Braz J Pharmaceut Sci*, *37*, 123-135.

Parise-Filho, R., Souza, T. M., Araujo, M. B., Fernandes, N. A. & Silveira, A. M. B. (2001). Chemical pharmaceutical analysis of oxamniquine and its pharmaceutical specialities. *Revista Brasileira Ciências Farmacêuticas*, *37*, 61-72.

Pérez del Villlar, L., Burguillo, F. J., Lopez-Aban, J. & Muro, A. (2012). Systematic review and meta-analysis of artemisinin based therapies for the treatment and prevention of schistosomiasis. *PloS One*, *7*, e45867.

Portela, J., et al. (2012). Antischistosomal Activity of Trioxaquines: In Vivo Efficacy and Mechanism of Action on Schistosoma mansoni. *PloS Negl Trop Dis*, *6*, e1474.

Sabah, A. A., Fletcher C., Webbe, G. & Dohenoff, M. J. (1986). Schistosoma mansoni, chemotherapy of infections of different ages. *Exp Parasitol*, *61*, 294-303.

Sarvel, A. K., Oliveira, A. A., Silva, A. R., Lima, A. C. L. & Katz, N. (2011). Evaluation of a 25-Year-Program for the Control of Schistosomiasis Mansoni in an Endemic Area in Brazil. *PLoS Negl Trop Dis*, *5*, e990.

Scholte, R. G. C., Carvalho, O. S., Malone, J. B., Utzinger, J. & Vounatsou, P. (2012). Spatial distribution of Biomphalaria spp., the intermediate host snails of Schistosoma mansoni, in Brazil. *Geospat Health*, *6*, S95-S101.

Schwartz E., Kozarsky, P., Wilson, M. & Cetron, M. (2005). Schistosome infection among river rafters on Omo River, Ethiopia. *J Travel Med*, *12*, 3–8.

Secor, W. E. (2006). Interactions between schistosomiasis and infection with HIV-1. *Parasite Immunol*, *28*, 597-603.

Silva, P. C. V. & Domingues, A. L. C. (2011). Aspectos epidemiológicos da esquistossomose hepatoesplênica no Estado de Pernambuco, Brasil. *Epidemiologia e Serviços de Saúde*, *20*, 327-336.

Silveira, A. C. (1989). Controle da Esquistossomose no Brasil. *Mem Inst Oswaldo Cruz*, *84*, 51-102.

Soares Magalhães, R. J., Barnett, A. G. & Clements, A. C. (2011). Geographical analysis of the role of water supply and sanitation in the risk of helminth infections of children in West Africa. *Proc Natl Acad Sci USA.108*, 20084-20089.

Soliman, R. & Hammouda, N.A. (1979). Synthesis of new mercaptotriazoles with potential antibilharzial activity. *J Pharma Sci*, *68*, 1377-1381.

Soliman, R., Mokhtar, H. N. & El-Sadany, S. K. (1984). Synthesis of new 8-(5-substituted amino-1, 3, 4-oxadiazol-2-yl) and 8-(5-substituted amino-1, 3, 4-thiadiazol-2-yl) methoxyquinolines with antibilharzial activity. *J Pharma Sci*, *73*, 403-405.

Souza, F. P. C., Vitorino, R. R., Costa, A. P., Faria, F. C., Santana, L. A. & Gomes, J. A. (2011). Esquistossomose mansônica, aspectos gerais, imunologia, patogênese e história natural. *Revista Brasileira de Clinica Medica*, *9*, 300-307.

Stelma, F. F., et al. (1995). Efficacy and side effects of praziquantel in an epidemic focus of Schistosoma mansoni. *Am J Trop Med Hyg*, *53*, 167-170.

Sweeney, T. R. (1981). The present status of malaria chemotherapy, mefloquine a novel antimalarial. *Med Res Reviews*, *1*, 181–201.

Thétiot-Laurent, S. A., Boissier, J., Robert, A. & Meunier, B. (2013). Schistosomiasis Chemotherapy. *Angew Chem Int*, *52*, 7936-7956.

Tukaebwa, E. M., et al. (2013). A Very High Infection Intensity of Schistosoma mansoni in a Ugandan Lake Victoria Fishing Community Is Required for Association with Highly Prevalent Organ Related Morbidity. *PLoS Negl Trop Dis*, *7*, e2268.

Uliana, S. R. & Barcinski, M. A. (2009). Repurposing for neglected diseases. *Science*, *326*, 935.

Utzinger, J. & Keiser, J. (2004). Schistosomiasis and soil-transmitted helminthiasis: common drugs for treatment and control. *Exp Opin Pharmacother*, *5*, 263-285.

Utzinger, J., Chollet, J., Tu, Z. W., Xiao, S. H. & Tanner, M. (2002). Comparative study of the effects of artemether and artesunate on juvenile and adult Schistosoma mansoni in experimentally infected mice. *Trans R Soc Trop Med Hyg*, *96*, 318-323.

Utzinger, J., Xiao, S. H., Keiser, J., Chen, M. G., Zheng, J. & Tanner, M. (2001). Current progress in the development and use of artemether for chemoprophylaxis of major human schistosome parasites. *Curr Med Chem*, *8*, 1841-1860.

Valencia, C. I., Catto, B. A., Webster, L. T., Jr. Barcelon, E. & Ofendo-Reyes R. (1994). Concentration time course of praziquantel in Filipinos with mild Schistosoma japonicum infection. *Southeast Asian J Trop Med Pub Health*, *25*, 409-414.

Veras, L. M., et al. (2012). Activity of epiisopiloturine against Schistosoma mansoni. *Curr Med Chem*, *19*, 2051-2058.

Verlinde C. L., et al. (2001). Glycolysis as a target for the design of new anti-trypanosome drugs. *Drug Resist Updates*, *4*, 50-65.

Webbe, G. & James, C. (1977). A comparison of the susceptibility to praziquantel of *Schistosoma haematobium*, *S. japonicum*, *S. mansoni*, *S. intercalatum* and *S. mattheei* in hamsters. *Parasitol Res*, *52*, 169-177.

WHO - World Health Organization (2006). Preventive chemotherapy in human helminthiasis: coordinated use of anthelminthic drugs in control interventions, a manual for health professionals and programme managers. Geneve.

WHO - World Health Organization. (2009). Elimination of schistosomiasis from low-transmission areas - Report of a WHO Informal Consultation. Geneve.

WHO - World Health Organization. (2010). *Schistosomiasis*, In: Media Centre - Fact sheets. Available at: http://www.who.int/mediacentre/factsheets/fs115/en/index.html

WHO - World Health Organization. (2010). First WHO report on neglected tropical diseases: working to overcome the global impact of neglected tropical diseases. Geneve: World Health Organization.

WHO - World Health Organization. (2002). *Medicina tradicional: necessidades crecientes y potencial*, In: Policy perspectives on medicine. Available at: http://whqlibdoc.who.int/hq/2002/who_edm_2002.4_spa.pdf

WHO – World Health Organization. (2013). *Schistosomiasis*. Available at: http://www.who.int/mediacentre/factsheets/fs115/en/(accessed on July 2013).

Wu, L. J., et al. (1995). Field aplication of artesunate in prophylaxis of schistosomiasis, na observation of 346 cases. *Chinese J Schistosomiasis Control*, *7*, 323-327.

Xiao, S. H. & Catto, B. A. (1989). In vitro and in vivo studies of the effect of artemether on Schistosoma mansoni. *Antimicrob Agents Chemother*, *33*, 1557-1562.

Xiao, S. H., Catto, B. A. & Webster, L. T. (1985). Effects of praziquantel on different developmental stages of Schistosoma mansoni in vitro and in vivo. *J Infect Dis*, *151*, 1130-1137.

Xiao, S. H., Hotez, P. J. & Tanner, M. (2000). Artemether, an effective new agent for chemoprophylaxis against schistosomiasis in China: its in vivo effect on the biochemical metabolism of the asian schistosome. *Southeast Asian J Trop Med Pub Health*, *31*, 724-732.

Xiao, S. H. (2005). Development of antischistosomal drugs in China, with particular consideration to praziquantel and the artemisinins. *Acta Trop*, *96*, 153-167.

Xiao, S .H., et al. (2007). In Vitro and In Vivo Activities of Synthetic Trioxolanes against Major Human Schistosome Species. *Antimicrob Agents Chemother*, *51*, 1440–1445.

Yue, W. J., You, J. Q. & Mei, J. Y. (1984). Effects of artemether on *Schistosoma japonicum* adult worms and ova. *Acta Pharmachol Sinica.*, *5*, 60-63.

Ziskind B. (2009). La bilharziose urinaire en ancienne Égypte. *Néphrologie & Thérapeutique*, *5*, 658–661.

In: Schistosomiasis
Editor: Adriana Erica Miele

ISBN: 978-1-63117-186-4

Chapter 4

Natural Products as a Source for Intermediate Host Control: Challenges and Advances in Schistosomiasis Research

***Lenita de Freitas Tallarico*[1,2,*]**
***and Ludmila Nakamura Rapado*[3]**
[1]Departamento de Biologia Funcional e Estrutural, Instituto de Biologia, Rua Charles Darwin, s/n Universidade Estadual de Campinas, Campinas, SP, Brazil
[2]Laboratório de Parasitologia, Instituto Butantan, São Paulo, SP, Brazil
[3]Unit for Drug Discovery, Departamento de Parasitologia, Instituto de Ciências Biomédicas, Universidade de São Paulo, São Paulo, SP, Brazil

Abstract

Schistosomiasis is an endemic parasitic disease that affects at least 240 million people, with more than 779 million at risk of infection. It is of considerable socioeconomic importance, with two main strategies for disease control. The goals of schistosomiasis control programmes are to

[*] Corresponding Author address: Departamento de Biologia Funcional e Estrutural, Instituto de Biologia, Rua Charles Darwin, s/n Universidade Estadual de Campinas, 13083-863, Campinas, SP, Brazil. E-mail: letallarico@gmail.com.

reduce the morbidity of human hosts by chemotherapy, and to manage the snail population in the lakes and freshwater sources of infected areas. The use of molluscicides has been considered by the World Health Organization as an appropriate method to prevent human infection in hazard areas. However, there are few effective products commercially available and the synthetic compound niclosamide is currently the best alternative. Researches on molluscicidal activity by natural products have been stimulated due to the high cost of synthetic pesticides, recurrent resistance of snails to these molecules and the low specificity of chemical compounds to snails. The marine and terrestrial environment represents a source of organisms that may contain useful products waiting to be discovered, which could be used in the treatment of several illnesses. In this Chapter, we will provide an overview of the current status of natural molluscicides and the perspectives for schistosomiasis control.

Keywords: Molluscicides, natural products, environment, ecology, schistosomiasis control programmes

Introduction

Schistosomiasis, also known as bilharziasis, is a tropical disease resulting from infection with parasitic trematode worms of the genus *Schistosoma*. Although the mortality rate is relatively low, this severe debilitating illness has affected millions of people to the present day [1].

According to the World Health Organization Report (WHO) [2], the main species of schistosomes that infect humans are listed in the chronological order in which they were first described: *Schistosoma haematobium* (1852), *S. japonicum* (1904), *S. mansoni* (1907), *S. intercalatum* (1934), and *S. mekongi* (1978). *S. malayensis* (1988) has also been described but its public-health significance is still undetermined, and *S. guianeensis* was only separated from *S. intercalatum* in 2003 [3]. There are two main schistosomiasis types, intestinal and urogenital, depending on the blood vessels of the mammalian hosts in which adult worms reside. Apart from *S. haematobium*, which is responsible for urogenital schistosomiasis, all the above cited species of fluke worms affect the intestine and liver [2]. Among the schistosome species, *S. haematobium*, *S. mansoni*, and *S. japonicum* cause the majority of human infections. The contamination requires no direct contact with intermediate hosts and the illness is acquired when free-swimming parasitic larvae (cercariae) penetrate the skin of people exposed to freshwater that contain infected snails [2, 4].

The species of freshwater snails are both medically and economically significant as intermediate hosts of the *Schistosoma* worms. The distribution of different species depends mainly on the ecology of the snail hosts. They may inhabit natural streams, ponds, lakes, reservoirs, and irrigation systems [4].

Each *Schistosoma* species has its own snails as a vector (see also chapter 2 of this book). The *Biomphalaria* genus serves as intermediate hosts of *S. mansoni* in Africa, the Arabian Peninsula, and the Americas. Snails of the genus *Bulinus* are the intermediate hosts of *S. haematobium* in Africa and the Eastern Mediterranean, as well as of *S. intercalatum* in Africa. *Oncomelania* is the *S. japonicum* intermediate host in China, the Philippines and Indonesia, and *Tricula* serves as the intermediate host of *S. mekongi* and is found in Laos and Cambodia [4, 5].

General Information about Intermediate Host Mollusks of Schistosomiasis

Among the mollusks, Gastropoda are the most diverse representatives of all classes of the Phylum Mollusca [6], with approximately 350 snail species with medical or veterinary importance. The majority of intermediate hosts for human *Schistosoma* belong to three genera, *Biomphalaria*, *Bulinus* and *Oncomelania*, which comprise freshwater snails [4].

The characteristics of several gastropods include the presence of a type of cover, along the entire body, formed by a tegument with special features, called mantle, given that its edge secretes a single-winged dorsal calcareous shell. Other characteristics include: a muscular foot flat ventral organ used for creeping feed, and an organ called radula [7]. The species can be identified by the shape of the shell. Snails can be separated into two main groups: aquatic snails that live under water and usually cannot survive elsewhere (this is the case of *Biomphalaria* and *Bulinus*), and amphibious snails, which adapted for living in and out of water (*Oncomelania*) [5].

The three important genera of snails, in general, were found in shallow water near the shores of lakes, ponds, marshes, streams and irrigation channels. They live on rocks, stones, concrete covered with algae, debris, aquatic plants and mud, in regions rich in decaying organic matter [5]. Snails require well-defined ecological conditions to thrive, an average temperature of 25°C is necessary to proliferate and reproduce, and some species resist long-term droughts. This explains the occurrence of schistosomiasis in locations where abundant water only occurs during rainy seasons. As a result, there is no transmission during dry seasons in these sites.

Biomphalaria and *Bulinus* are aquatic organisms that belong to the family Planorbidae. They are simultaneous hermaphrodites, possessing both male and female organs and being capable of self or cross-fertilization. One single specimen can invade and populate a new habitat. The egg masses are laid at intervals in batches of 5–40, each batch being enclosed in a mass of gelatinous material. Temperature and food availability are among the most important limiting factors for this species [5]. *Oncomelania* belongs to the family Pomatiopsidae [8]. These snails have separate sexes, the eggs are singly spawned and laid on the water margin. This genus is capable of living for several years [5].

Prevention and Disease Control

Studies regarding schistosomiasis control date back to 1919 [9], and since the 1950s, the WHO has recommended successive strategies for schistosomiasis control on a global scale [10-18].

Initially, in 1950, among the measures for schistosomiasis control, two were the priorities: discovery of molluscicides with prolonged activity and restricted to the target species at low concentrations, with minimal environmental impact, low cost and easy application; and discovery of effective and safe chemotherapeutic drugs. In the 60s the intermediate hosts combat was recognized as the most effective single measure in schistosomiasis control, since no drug or other control measures were promising [18].

In 1970, WHO reported that patient's treatment, associated with the snails control gave faster results on the incidence, prevalence and transmission intensity of the disease when compared to the use of molluscicides as the single measure of control. However, the importance of the use of a molluscicide was reiterated as well as the recommendation to develop new and improved molluscicides aiming at a maximum effect and minimum cost [18].

In the 80s, due to the development of simple and fast quantitative diagnostic methods, as well as the pharmaceutical industry investment in the development of safe and effective drugs, especially Praziquantel, there was a change in the approach of schistosomiasis control. WHO has put the human host as the center of attention in the transmission disease control and the molluscicides application became an auxiliary measure in this scheme. In

1985, the decrease in morbidity was the goal of control programs. From the 2000s, schistosomiasis control has been done in an integrated manner to the Geohelminths, with treatment of high-risk groups without prior individual diagnosis. Due to lack of effective molluscicides, this control method is no prioritized, but is used in places of high endemicity for it is considered the only effective measure to reduce transmission of the disease in the short term [18, 19].

At this moment there is no consensus in the scientific community about the best control strategy for combating schistosomiasis [20]. However, it is known that no single method is able to control the transmission of the illness, requiring a combination of control measures, which must be held for the long term in order to interrupt the transmission cycle between *Schistosoma*, the mammalian host, and the snail vectors [21-23].

Prevention and control of schistosomiasis are primarily based on the treatment of individual patients, together with three large scale schemes: (i) environmental management, control of intermediate hosts with molluscicides or biological control; (ii) improvement of public health services, provision of safe water and sanitation; (iii) behavioral change through health education and community participation in adopting preventive measures, such as individual protection to prevent the cercariae skin penetration. Altogether these measures are the most effective control on the medium and long terms. However, in theory, one efficient method is difficult to perform in large endemic areas [2, 4, 24, 25, 26]. According to Fenwick and Savioli [27] the implementation of integrated programs with the treatment of patients with Praziquantel and employment of molluscicide are still the best options for schistosomiasis control.

This chapter will address the study and analysis of compounds from plants and marine organisms as potential molluscicides for controlling snail hosts of the three main species that cause human schistosomiasis.

History of Molluscicides in Schistosomiasis Control

Mollusks play an important role in the transmission of the disease. An intense multiplication and the formation of an infective stage of *Schistosoma* occur inside snail hosts. Strategies involving their control are recommended to reduce disease transmission, since snails are the most vulnerable organisms in the schistosomiasis life cycle and their disposal prevents infection of people in contact with water in hazardous areas [28-30].

According to the WHO, a molluscicide compound is considered optimal when the substance at a low concentration eliminates all mollusk life cycle stages, from the embryo to the adult, for snails living under given environmental conditions.

The substance must be low cost, stable to store, independently of temperature and solar irradiation, should not present a risk in transportation, handling and application, should not suffer decomposition in water and soil, and must provide selective lethal action to snails, while being harmless to humans, pets, fish and plants [11, 12, 16].

The first chemical molluscicides, used between 1913 and 1915, were derived from calcium and copper [31, 32]. Subsequently, several chemicals (about 20,000) have been evaluated for molluscicidal activity. Among them, pentachlorophenol and its salts, sodium and copper pentachlorophenate, were identified as highly lethal to mollusks, interfering in vital enzymatic processes. However, their toxicity to several organisms prevented their use on a large scale [11, 14].

Nowadays, niclosamide (2',5-dichloro-4'-nitrosalicylanilide) (Figure 1) is the molluscicide recommended by WHO for use in schistosomiasis control programmes [17]. However, this compound is toxic to several other species of mollusks, fish and other aquatic organisms, and prolonged use causes damage to terrestrial and aquatic plants. Moreover, its production cost is high, the compound rapidly decomposes under sunlight exposure and its application does not prevent surviving snails from starting recolonization, therefore it requires frequent reapplications, which would result in the undesired selection of resistant populations [33-36].

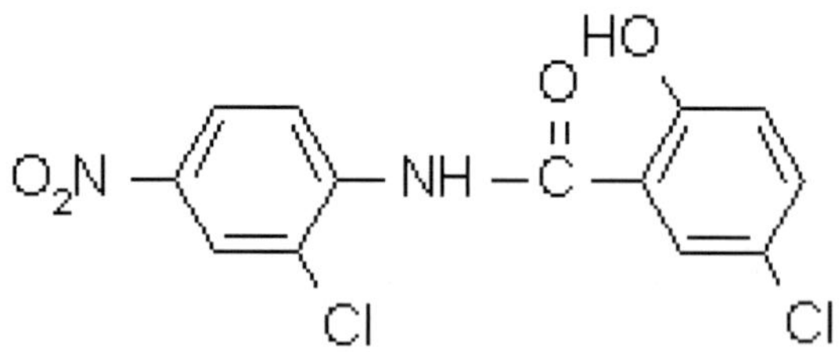

Figure 1. Chemical structure of Niclosamide (2'5-dichloro-4'-nitro-salicylanilide). Molecular weight: 327.12; chemical formula: $C_{13}H_8LC_2N_2O_4$.

Natural Products as Agents of Schistosomiasis Control

The lack of one single effective method for disease control, the high cost of the methods, the inefficiency of currently available synthetic molluscicides and the quest for alternative non-polluting solutions aiming towards environmental preservation encourage the research of natural molluscicides [12, 36-44].

Based on knowledge of the molluscicidal activity of an organism, different methodologies can be developed to obtain active compounds. The choice depends on the information available about the species to be studied. In general, the search for active compounds is carried out by evaluating the activity of compounds that already were isolated *versus* crude extracts, followed by chemical isolation, in which each step is associated with monitoring the molluscicidal activity of each fraction; and by chemical profiling obtained by High Performance Liquid Chromatography (HPLC) and Nuclear Magnetic Resonance (NMR). These methods allow the identification and discovery of new molecules with potential biological activity [45, 46].

Studies of marine and plant species have been conducted according to the WHO specifications for chemical molluscicides [11, 12, 16], which define a molluscicide as feasible when it presents toxic effects in adult mollusks in concentrations less than or equal to 20 mg/mL of the isolated compound and less than or equal to 100 mg/mL of crude extract. The active compound should be preferentially extracted with water and remain active when physical and chemical changes occur, such as changes in pH, sunlight and temperature [38, 47].

Plants with molluscicidal activity have been studied since 1930 and this discovery allowed the use of some species in control programs. Archibald [48] used the fruits of species *Balanites aegyptiaca* and *Balanites maughamii* in aqueous extract, with the resulting composition containing saponin and isobutylamide spirostane, which killed *Biomphalaria* and *Bulinus*, miracidium and cercariae of *S. mansoni* in Sudan [38].

Archibald [48] and Anantaraman [49] recommended that *B. aegyptiaca* were planted around the schistosomiasis endemic areas, because the fruit of said tree falling in the water would inhibit the snail population without changing the drinking water. The species *Ambrosia maritima* and *Sapindus saponaria* were employed in the irrigated fields with the same purpose [50, 51].

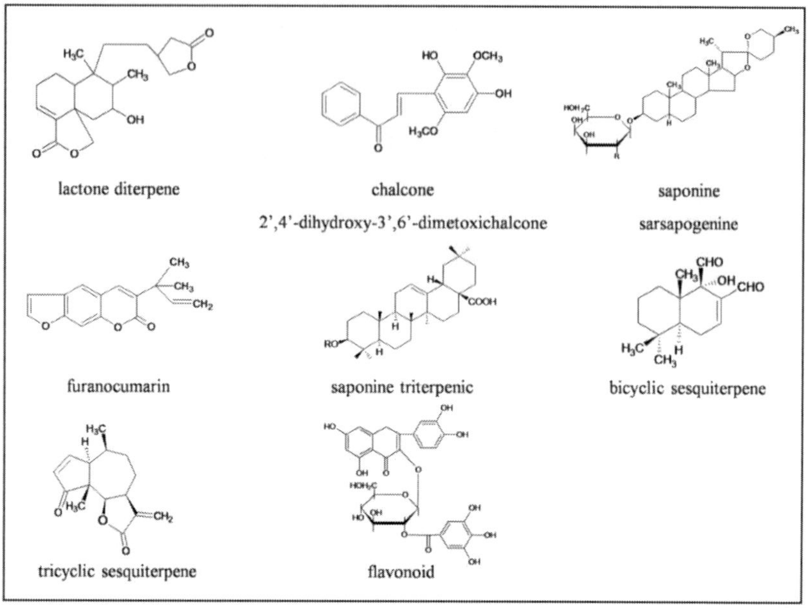

Figure 2. Chemical structure of the first compounds described with molluscicidal activity.

Henderson and collaborators [52], during a preliminary isolation and identification of plant compounds with molluscicidal activity, obtained active substances in concentrations less than or equal to 1 mg/mL. The first identified compound belonged to the class of saponins, being triterpenoids and spirostane. They subsequently identified coumarins and furanocoumarins, flavonoids, sesquiterpenes quinolizidine, alkaloids, lactones diterpenes and tannins (Figure 2). Among these, tannins and saponins were the most promising.

Saponins are soluble in water and present toxicity and hemolytic action for *B. glabrata* (LC_{90} 1.5 μg/mL). However, they are toxic to fish and aquatic vertebrates at low concentrations, due to interference with their respiratory processes, causing paralysis in the function of the gills. The tannins, although being easily extracted with water and presenting low toxicity to aquatic organisms, have reduced molluscicidal effect when compared to saponin (LC_{90} 50 μg/mL in *B. glabrata*) [53, 54].

Researches have been conducted in order to discover natural compounds with molluscicidal activity and lower environmental impact than that caused by niclosamide. Table 1 presents some of these compounds.

Table 1. Molluscicidal activity and toxicity of some isolated natural compounds on intermediate hosts of schistosomiasis

Compound/Substance	Species	Origin	Activity Adult	Embryos	Toxicity	Ref
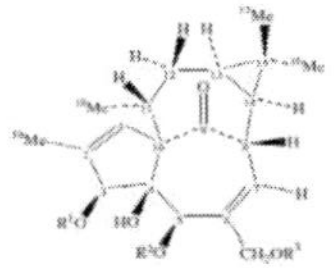 N-(2-aminobenzoyl) anthranilic ester	*Euphorbia cornigera* Boiss	Plant	LC_{50} 11.4-75.4 µg/mL in *B. glabrata*	No activity	Not evaluated	[55]
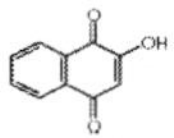 lausone 2-hydroxy-[1,4]naphthoquinone	*Euphorbia cornigera* Boiss	Plant	LC_{90} 4.2-92.7 µg/mL in *B. glabrata*	Not evaluated	toxic to *Artemia salina*	[16]
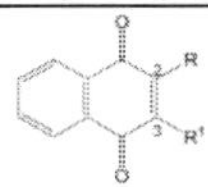 derivated compounds of [1,4] naphthoquinone	*Euphorbia cornigera* Boiss	Plant	LC_{90} 4.2-92.7 µg/mL in *B. glabrata*	Not evaluated	toxic to *Artemia salina*	[16]
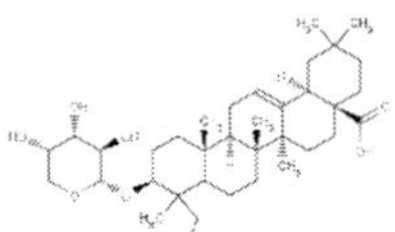 leontoside A	*Cephalaria ambrosioides* Sibth. & Sm.	Plant	LC_{100} 5.4 µg/mL in *B. glabrata*	Not evaluated	Not evaluated	[56]

Table 1. (Continued)

Compound/Substance	Species	Origin	Activity Adult	Embryos	Toxicity	Ref
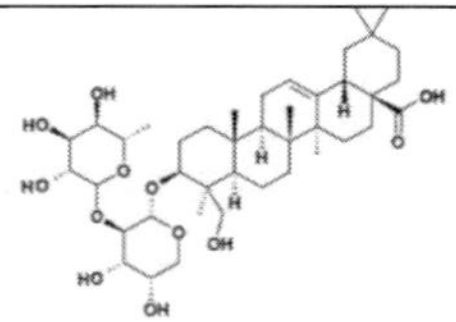 calopanax A	*Cephalaria ambrosioides* Sibth. & Sm.	Plant	LC_{100}6.2 μg/mL in *B. glabrata*	Not evaluated	Not evaluated	[56]
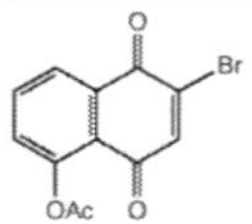 2-bromo-5-acetoxy-1,4- naphthoquinone	*Cephalaria ambrosioides* Sibth. & Sm	Plant	LC_{90} 2.2 μg/mL in *B. glabrata*	Not evaluated	Not evaluated	[57]
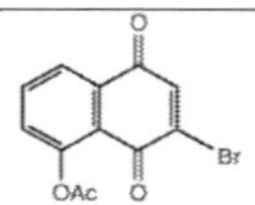 3-bromo-5- acetoxy-1,4- naphthoquinone	*Cephalaria ambrosioides* Sibth. & Sm	Plant	LC_{90} 1.6 μg/mL in *B. glabrata*	Not evaluated	Not evaluated	[57]
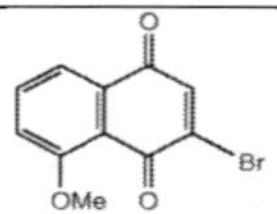 3-bromo-5-metox-1,4 naphthoquinone	*Cephalaria ambrosioides* Sibth. & Sm	Plant	LC_{90} 1.4 μg/mL in *B. glabrata*	Not evaluated	Not evaluated	[57]
lectines D glucose/ mannose binding – proteins	*Cratylia floribunda* Benth.	Plant	LC_{90} 50.3 μg/mL in *B. glabrata*	Not evaluated	Toxic to *Artemia salina*	[58]
lectines glucose/manose binding protein	*Diolcea guianensis* Benth.	Plant	LC_{90} 41.μg/mL in *B. glabrata*	Not evaluated	Toxic to *Artemia salina*	[58]

Compound/Substance	Species	Origin	Activity Adult	Embryos	Toxicity	Ref
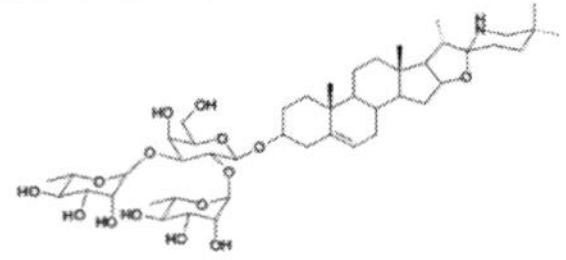 Solamargine	*Solanum sisymbriifolium* Lam	Plant	LC_{100} 148 µg /mL in *B. pfeifferi*	Not evaluated	toxic to fishes, insects, larvae	[59]
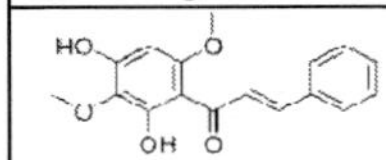 2,4-dihydroxy 3',6'- dimethoxy chalcone	*Polygonum senegalense*Meisn	Plant	LC_{100} 10 µg/mL in *B. glabrata*	Not evaluated	Not evaluated	[60]
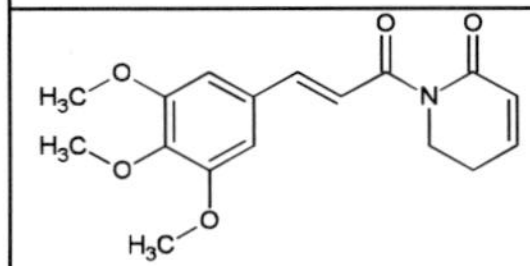 Piplartine	*Piper tuberculatum* Jacq	Plant	LC_{90} 6.94 µg/mL in *B. glabrata*	LC_{90} 0.99-4.35 µg/mL	*Daphnia similis* 48 h EC_{50} 7.32 µg/mL [6.93–7.69] *Danio rerio* 48 h LC_{50} 1.69 µg/mL [1.61–1.77]	[35]
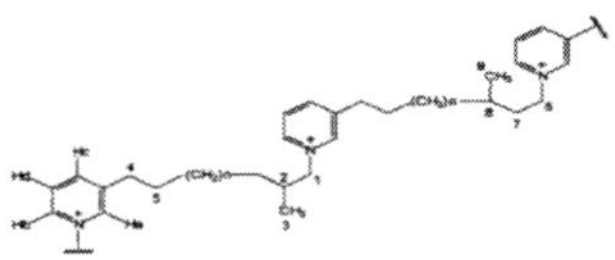 Halitoxin	*Amphimedon viridis*	Sponge	LC_{50} 20 µg/mL in *B. glabrata*	No activity	Not evaluated	[37]
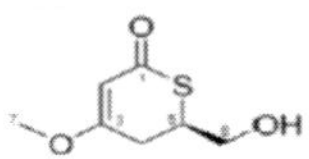 Thiopalmyrone	*Oscillatoria* spp	Cyanobacteria	LC_{50} 8.3 µM in *B. glabrata*	Not evaluated	Not evaluated	[61]

Table 1. (Continued)

Compound/Substance	Species	Origin	Activity Adult	Embryos	Toxicity	Ref
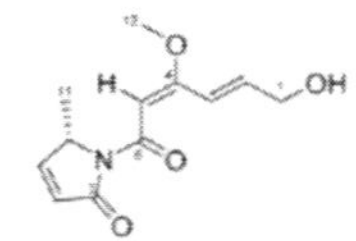 Palmyrrolinone	*Hormoscilla* spp	Cyanobac teria	LC_{50} 6. μM in *B. glabrata*	Not evaluated	Not evaluated	[61]
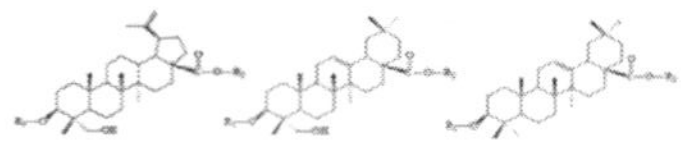 Saponines	*Pulsatilla chinensis (Bunge) Regel*	Plant	LC_{95} 2.94μg/mL in *Oncomelania hupensis*	Not evaluated	32 mg/L for 72 h, killed 100% of *Danio rerio*.	[62]
Alkaloids	*Eomecon chionantha*	Plant	LC_{100} 2.5 μg/mL in *Oncomelania hupensis*	Not evaluated	Not evaluated	[63]
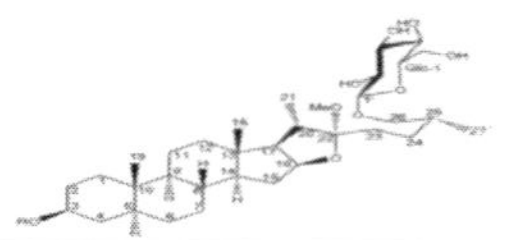	*Yucca desmettiana*	Plant	LC_{100} at 6 μg/mL in *B. alexandrina*	Not evaluated	Not evaluated	[64]
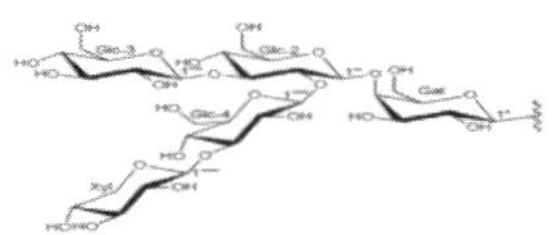	*Yucca desmettiana*	Plant	LC_{100} at 11 μg/mL in *B. alexandrina*	Not evaluated	Not evaluated	[64]

However, until now, no effective products have been discovered because it was not possible to find one isolated compound that acts only on the target snail and due to difficulties during compound synthesis in order to produce quantities for world-scale use.

The family Euphorbiaceae comprises species that produce latex, and it is composed by terpenes with molluscicidal (100% lethality to *B. glabrata* at 1.5 μg/mL) and schistosomicidal activities [65-67]. Among the compounds listed in Table 1, the species of the genus *Euphorbia* are the most investigated. These investigations include toxicity analyses and field studies. A study in endemic areas showed that the use of *Euphorbia splendens* var. *hislopii* (concentration of 5μg/mL) latex, applied twice with an interval of two weeks, was more effective than niclosamide [68]. However, the latex of the *Euphorbia* species is generally toxic to aquatic organisms and does not eliminate *Biomphalaria* embryos, impeding the snail's elimination [39, 69].

The piplartine amide is widely studied as an anti-parasitic agent (leishmanicidal trypanocidal and schistosomicidal) and antitumor agent [70-74]; it is also a promising molluscicide, since it causes mortality to all the developmental stages of *B. glabrata* and induces less environmental toxicity than niclosamide [42].

The marine environment presents great biodiversity, however, the acquired knowledge on organisms that inhabit this ecosystem is still scarce, especially in deep waters, where exploration has only recently begun and new species are discovered every year. Marine organisms have demonstrated to be among the most promising sources of new bioactive compounds for the treatment of different human diseases [75, 76], such as in anti-parasitic applications against several organisms [77,-80]. Currently, only studies on red algae *Liagora farinosa* and sponge *Amphimedon viridis* (halitoxin) have demonstrated they could be potential sources of secondary metabolites for population control of intermediate host snails of schistosomiasis [44].

The mechanisms by which natural compounds kill snails and embryos or exert teratogenic action are still unclear. The molluscicide action requires further investigation in order to unravel possible mechanisms of action for toxicity against the snails.

Toxicity Studies of the Active Compounds

After obtaining a compound with molluscicidal action, WHO [47] recommends performing toxicity assays on vertebrates and invertebrates in order to evaluate potential harmful effects in humans, animals and plants. In this way, ecotoxicological assays are performed to estimate the impact that a chemical compound causes to the ecosystem. For these analyses, the use of a representative species with ecological significance for the environment is a necessary tool for monitoring chemical compounds. Furthermore, the use of diverse organisms of different trophic levels is essential [81, 82].

Some organisms, such as micro-crustaceans (*Daphnia magna* and *Ceriodaphnia dubia*), algae (*Pseudokirchneriella subcapitata* and *Chlorella vulgaris*), and fish (*Danio rerio* and *Pimephales promelas*), are considered good experimental models for ecotoxicological assays, since they have been validated and standardized through constant use in toxicity assays [83-89].

Although many compounds have been studied as possible molluscicides (Table 1), at this moment, there are very few data on their toxicity towards standardized organisms. For a first compound toxicity analysis assays the use of several organisms is necessary. The studies of Camara et al. [16] and Santos et al. [58] demonstrate that plant compounds *Euphorbia cornigera*, *Cratylia floribunda* and *Diolcea guianensis* were toxic to marine crustacean *Artemia salina*. But it should be emphasized the importance of assays that employ native species with ecological significance for aquatic environment where the molluscicide will be release. Rapado et al. [42] suggest the use of two standardized species for this purpose, the microcrustacean *Daphnia similis* and the fish *Danio rerio*. The lack of information about toxicity in aquatic organisms makes evident the need for implementation of ecotoxicological assays for the establishment of new substances.

Preventive measures, especially those aimed at controlling the snails, directly affect the environment and should be in consonance with environmental legislation in regions that are transmission foci.

Perspectives in the Development of Molluscicides from Natural Products

Until now, natural compounds were the source of choice for developing new drugs for parasite control. However, combating the intermediate hosts has been recently discussed as an important tool for controlling the illness, with natural products being considered as possible targets for obtaining active molecules. In this context, the almost totally unexplored marine biodiversity is a potential ecosystem for obtaining new chemical structures that have not yet been described.

As mentioned above, several compounds show molluscicidal activity, some being considered promising since they are active against all snails life stages (from embryos to adults). But the feasibility of using these compounds is questioned because there are no studies that report their impact on the environment. It is therefore necessary to implement environmental impact assessments of new compounds in organisms standardized for this purpose. In addition, another approach must be taken into consideration, the field studies, required for the validation and reproducibility of the tests when the compound is released into a given freshwater source.

Data presented here indicated that molluscicide action requires a deep investigation in order to unravel possible mechanisms of action for toxicity against snail vectors, since neither niclosamide, despite being used since the 80's, has its mechanisms of action elucidated. It is believed that the snails death exposed to chemicals possibly occur due to changes in more than one physiological system. Rapado et al. [42] and Miyasato et al. [44] observed that adult snails released hemolymph when subjected to crude or fractionated extracts. This can be associated to reduction of the heart rate, swelling of the tissues due to alteration of cellular water balance; all of these lead to rupture of the external membranes and to the release of mollusks hemolymph through the hemal pore [47, 90].

Normally, the effects of natural compounds towards embryos are more intense than on adult snails, but first of all, the substance(s) must cross through biological membranes. Disturbances in these stages can lead to arrested development and inviability of the developing organism [42, 44, 91]. This sensitivity is assigned to intense cell proliferation activity in the early developmental stages [92]. Substances that induce embryotoxicity can lead to decrease viability of exposed eggs and reduce the snail population in an infested region [39].

Another focus of study is the synthesis of structural analogues of the compounds with high toxicity, in the search for molecules that allow the reduction of toxicity while still preserving the molluscicidal activity.

Despite the low index of the schistosomiasis reduction, some issues should be taken into consideration besides prioritizing patient treatment and parasite control. Several studies report that one possibility is to control illness prevalence levels. However, this control would only be effective with integrated preventive measures. Nowadays, despite the existence of schistosomiasis vaccine candidates and chemotherapeutic programmes, the control of intermediate host snails through the discovery of new natural compounds and synthesis of active molecule has been viable for reducing the incidence of the disease, and in the case of Japan (the only winning story) to complete eradicate the disease.

References

[1] World Health Organization (2011). *Weekly epidemiological record.* World Health Organization, Geneva, v. 9, n. 86, 73-80.

[2] World Health Organization (2013). *Strategic Plan 2012–2020. Schistosomiasis: Progress report 2001–2011 and Strategic plan 2012–2020,* World Health Organization, Geneva, 1-80.

[3] Kane, RA; Southgate, VR; Rollinson, D; Littlewood, DTJ; Lockyer, AE; Pagès, JR; Tchuem Tchuenté, LA; Jourdane, J. (2003). A phylogeny based on three mitochondrial genes supports the division of *Schistosoma intercalatum* into two separate species. *Parasitology*, 127(2): 131-137.

[4] Gryseels, B; Polman, K; Cerinx, J; Kestens, L (2006). Human schistosomiasis. *Lancet* 368:1106-1118.

[5] World Health Organization (1997). Freshwater snails Intermediate hosts of schistosomiasis and foodborne trematode infections. In: *Vector control: Methods for use by individuals and communities.* World Health Organization, Geneva, 337-356.

[6] Barnes, RTD (1990). The Mollusk. In: *Zoology invertebrate.* 4ed., Livraria Rocca, São Paulo, 277-278.

[7] Barnes, RSK; Calow, P; Olive, JW (1995). *Os invertebrados: uma nova síntese.* São Paulo, Atheneu, 136-155.

[8] Bouchet, P; Rocroi, JP. (2005). Classification and Nomenclator of Gastropod Families. *Malacologia* 47 (1-2): 397.

[9] Annon (1919). Bilharziasis: its prevention and treatment. *Lancet* 193:1032.

[10] World Health Organization (1953). WHO expert committee on bilharziasis: first report. Geneva. *Technical report series*, 53.

[11] World Health Organization (1961). Molluscicides. *World Health Organ Technical Report Serie*, 214: 1-59.

[12] World Health Organization (1965) Molluscicide screening and evaluation. In: *Bulletin of the World Health Organization*, Geneva 33: 567–581.

[13] World Health Organization (1967) Epidemiology and Control of Schistosomiasis. Report of a WHO Expert Committee. Geneva, *Technical report series*, 372.

[14] World Health Organization (1973). Schistosomiasis control. *Report of a World Health Organization Expert Committee*. Geneva, 515: 1-47.

[15] World Health Organization (1980) Epidemiology and control of schistosomiasis. *World Health Organ Technical Report Serie*, 649: 1-76.

[16] World Health Organization (1985). The control of schistosomiasis. *World Health Organ Technical Report Series*, 728: 1-113.

[17] World Health Organization (1993). The control of role of schistosomiasis. Second report of WHO Expert Committee. *World Health Organ Technical Report Series*, 830: 1-86.

[18] World Health Organization (2002). Prevention and Control of Schistosomiasis and soil-transmitted Helminthiasis: Report of a WHO Expert Committee. Geneva, *Technical Report Series*, 912.

[19] Carvalho, OS; Amaral, RS; Dutra, LV; Scholte, RGC; Guerra MAM. (2008). Distribuição espacial de *Biomphalaria glabrata*, *B. straminea* e *B. tenagophila*, hospedeiros intermediários de *Schistosoma mansoni* no Brasil. In: *Schistosoma mansoni* e Esquistossomose: uma visão multidisciplinar. 20ª ed. Rio de Janeiro, Editora Fiocruz, 394-418.

[20] Rollinson, D; Knopp, S; Levitz, S; Stothard, JR; Tchuem Tchuenté, LA; Garba, A; Mohammed, KA; Schur, N; Person, B; Colley, DG; Utzinger, J. (2013). Time to set the agenda for schistosomiasis elimination. *Acta Trop*. 128(2): 423-440.

[21] Gray, DJ; McManus, DP; Li, Y; Williams, GM; Bergquist, R; Ross, AG. (2010). Schistosomiasis elimination: lessons from the past guide the future. *Lancet Infect. Dis*. 10:733-736.

[22] Zhang, Z; Jiang, Q .(2011). Schistosomiasis elimination. *Lancet Infect. Dis*., 11 (5): 345.

[23] Chimbari, MJ. (2012). Enhancing Schistosomiasis Control Strategy for Zimbabwe: Building on Past Experiences. *J. Paras. Res*., 2012: 353768.

[24] Fenwick, A; Webster, JP. (2006). Schistosomiasis - challenges for control, treatment and drug resistance. *Curr. Opinion Infect. Dis*, 19: 577-582.

[25] Steinmann, P; Keiser, J; Bos, R; Tanner, M; Utzinger, J. (2006) Schistosomiasis and water resources development: systematic review, meta-analysis, and estimates of people at risk. *Lancet Infect. Dis*. 6: 411-425.

[26] Ministério da Saúde, 2008. Algumas considerações sobre o controle da esquistossomose. In: *Vigilância e Controle de Moluscos de Importância Epidemiológica.* Secretaria da Vigilância da Saúde. Ministério da Saúde. 2ª Edição, 133-134.

[27] Fenwick, A; Savioli, L. (2011). Schistosomiasis elimination. *Lancet Infect. Dis.*, 11(5): 346-347.

[28] Camara, CA; Silva, TM; da-Silva, TG; Martins, RM; Barbosa, TP; Pinto, AC; Vargas MD (2008). Molluscicidal activity of 2-hydroxy- 1,4 naphthoquinone and derivatives. *Ann. Acad. Bras. Cienc.* 80(2):329-33.

[29] Lardans, V; Dissous, C (1998). Snail control strategies for reduction of schistosomiasis transmission. *Parasitol. Today*. 14(10): 413-417.

[30] World Health Organization (1984). Report of informal consultation on research on the biological control of snail intermediated hosts. *Bulletin of the World Health Organization*, 41.

[31] Mccullough, F; Mott KE(1983). The role of molluscicides in schistosomiasis control. *Bulletin World Health Organization*, 1-13.

[32] Webbe, G (1987). Molluscicide in the control of schistosomiasis. In: Mott, KE. (Ed.). *Plant Molluscicides*. Chichester: John Wiley, 1-26.

[33] Abreu, FC; Goulart, MOF; Brett, A M O (2002). Detection of the damage caused to DNA by niclosamide using an electrochemical DNA-biosensor. *Biosens. Bioelectron.*, 17(11-12): 913-919.

[34] Giovanelli, A; Silva, CL; Medeiros, L; Vasconcellos, MC (2002). The molluscicidal activity of niclosamide (Bayluscide WP70®) on *Melanoides tuberculata* (Thiaridae), a snail associated with habitats of *Biomphalaria glabrata* (Planorbidae). *Mem. Inst. Oswaldo Cruz,* 97(5): 743-745.

[35] Pointier, JP; Giboda, M (1999). The case for biological control of snail intermediate hosts of *Schistosoma mansoni. Parasitol. Today*, 15(10): 395-397.

[36] World Health Organization (1992). The role of mollusciciding in Schistosomiasis control. *Bulletin of the World Health Organization*, 107.

[37] Bezerra, JCB; Silva, IA; Ferreira, HD; Ferri, PH; Santos, SC (2002) Molluscicidal activity against *Biomphalaria glabrata* of Brazilian Cerrado medicinal plants. *Fitoterapia* 73: 428-430.

[38] Kloos, H; Mccullough, F S (1982). Plant molluscicides. *J. Medical Plant. Res.,* 46: 195-209.

[39] Oliveira-Filho, EC, Geraldino BR, Coelho DR, De-Carvalho RR, Paumgartten FJr (2010) Comparative toxicity of Euphorbia milii latex

and synthetic molluscicides to *Biomphalaria glabrata* embryos. *Chemosphere* 81: 218–227.

[40] Oliveira-Filho, EC; Paumgartten, JR (2000). Toxicity of *Euphorbia milii* látex and niclosamide to snails and nontarget aquatic species. *Ecotoxicol. Environ. Saf.*, 46:342-350.

[41] Rapado LN, Nakano E, Ohlweiler FP, Kato MJ, Yamaguchi LF, Pereira CAB, Kawano T (2010) Molluscicidal and ovicidal activities of plant extracts of the Piperaceae on Biomphalaria glabrata (Say, 1818). *J. Helminthol.* 85(1): 66-72.

[42] Rapado, LN; Pinheiro, AS; Lopes POMV; Fokoue, HH, Scotti, MT, Marques, JV; Ohlweiler, FP; Borrely, SI; Pereira, CA; Kato, MJ; Nakano, E; Yamaguchi, LF (2013). Schistosomiasis Control Using Piplartine against *Biomphalaria glabrata* at Different Developmental Stages. *Plos Negl. Trop. Dis.* 7(6): e2251.

[43] Singh, SK; Yadav, RP; Singh, A (2010). Molluscicides from some common medicinal plants of eastern Uttar Pradesh, India. *J. Appl. Toxicol.*, 30 (1): 1-7.

[44] Miyasato, PA; Kawano, T; Freitas, JC; Berlinck, RGS; Nakano, E; Tallarico, LF (2012) Molluscicidal activity of some marine substances against the snail *Biomphalaria glabrata* (Mollusca, Planorbidae). *Parasitol Res.* 110(5): 1873-1879.

[45] Hostettman, K; Queiroz, EF; Vieira, PC (2003). A procura dos princípios ativos. In: *Princípios ativos de plantas superiores.* São Carlos: EDUFSCar, 43-58.

[46] Falkenberg, MB; Santos, RI; Simões, CMO (2007). Introdução à análise fitoquímica. In: *Farmacognosia da planta ao medicamento.* 6ª ed. Porto Alegre, UFRGS, 229-262.

[47] World Health Organization (1983). *Report of the scientific working group on plant molluscicides.* World Health Organization, Geneva, 12: 1–11.

[48] Archibald, R G (1933). The use of the fruit of the tree *Balanites aegyptiaca* in the control of schistosomiasis in the country-region Sudan. *Trans. R Soc. Trop. Med. Hyg.*, 27: 207.

[49] Anantaraman, M (1995). Biological control of aquatic snail. *Indian J. Vet. Res.*, 25: 65-67.

[50] Kloos, H; Mccullough, FS (1987). Plant with recognized molluscicidal activity. In: Mott, KE (Ed.). *Plant molluscicides.* Chichester: John Wiley, 45-108.

[51] Jurberg, P; De Vasconcellos, M. C.; Mendes, N. M. (1989). Plants used as molluscacides - a critical-view. *Mem. Inst. Oswaldo Cruz*, 84: 76-83.

[52] Henderson, TO; Farnsworth, N; Myers, T (1987). Biochemistry of recognized molluscicidal compounds of plant origin. In: Mott, KE (Ed.) *Plant molluscicides*. Chichester: John Wiley, 109-130.

[53] Costa, SS; Mors, W (1981). Amides of *Ottonia corcovadensis*. *Phytochemistry*, 20(6): 1305-1307.

[54] Hostettmann, K; Marston, A (1987). Plant molluscicide research. In: Mott, KE (Ed.) *Plant molluscicides.* Chichester: John Wiley, 299-320.

[55] Baloch, I B; Baloch, M K; Baloch, AK (2009). Bio-active compounds from *Euphorbia cornigera* Boiss. *Eur. J. Med. Chem.*, 44: 3188-3194.

[56] Pasi, S; Aligiannis, N; Pratsinis, H; Skaltsounis, AL; Chinou, IB (2009). Biologically active triterpenoids from *Cephalaria ambrosioides. Planta Med.*, 75: 163-167.

[57] Ribeiro, KA; Carvalho, CM; Molina, MT; Lima, EP; López-Montero, E; Reys, JR; Oliveira, MB; Pinto, AV; Santana, AE; Goulart, MO (2009). Activities of naphthoquinones against *Aedes aegypti* (Linnaeus, 1762) (Diptera: Culicidae), vector of dengue and *Biomphalaria glabrata* (Say, 1818), intermediate host of *Schistosoma mansoni. Acta Trop.*, 111: 44-50.

[58] Santos, AF; Cavada, BS; Rocha, BA; Nascimento, KS; Sant'Ana, AE (2010).Toxicity of some glucose/mannose-binding lectins to *Biomphalaria glabrata* and *Artemia salina. Bioresour. Technol.*, 101: 794-798.

[59] Bagalwa, JJ; Voutquenne-Nazabadioko, L; Sayagh, C; Bashwira, AS (2010). Evaluation of the biological activity of the molluscicidal fraction of *Solanum sisymbriifolium* against non target organisms. *Fitoterapia*, 81: 767-771.

[60] Adewunmi, CO; Ogungbamila, FO; Oluwadiya, O (1987). Molluscicidal activities of some synthetic chalcones. *Planta Med.*, 53(1): 110-112.

[61] Pereira, AR; Etzbach, L; Engene, N; Muller, R; Gerwick, WH (2011). Molluscicidal metabolites from an assemblage of Palmyra Atoll cyanobacteria. *J. Nat. Prod.*, 74: 1175-1181.

[62] Chen, YQ; Xu, QM; Liu, YL; Li, XR; Yang, SL; Zhuge, HX (2012). Laboratory Evaluation of the Molluscicidal Activity of *Pulsatilla Chinensis* (Bunge) Regel Saponins against the Snail *Oncomelania hupensis. Biomed. Environ. Sci.*, 25(2): 224-229.

[63] Peng, F; Liu, M; Huang, Q; Liu, N; Yang, H; Sun, H; Hu, Q; Feng, F; Jiang, C (2011). Molluscicidal effect of *Eomecon chionantha* alkaloids

against *Oncomelania hupensis* snails. *Southeast Asian J. Trop. Med. Public Health,* 42(2): 289-296.

[64] Diab, Y; Ioannou, E; Emam, A; Vagias, C; Roussis, V (2012). Desmettianosides A and B, bisdesmosidic furostanol saponins with molluscicidal activity from *Yucca desmettiana. Steroids*, 77(6): 686-90.

[65] Baptista, DF; Vasconcellos, MC; Lopes, FE; Silva, IP; Schall VT (1994). Perspectives of using *Euphorbia splendens* as a molluscicide in schistosomiasis control programs. *Southeast Asian J. Trop. Med. Public Health*, 25(3): 419-424.

[66] De-Carvalho, RR; Maldonado Júnior, A; Oliveira Filho, EC; Ribeiro, AC; Paumgartten, FJ; Rey, L (1998). Effects of *Euphorbia milii* latex on *Schistosoma mansoni* eggs, miracidia and cercariae. *Mem. Inst. Oswaldo Cruz,* 93, Supl 1: 235-237.

[67] Schall, VT; de Vasconcellos, MC; de Souza, CP; Baptista, DF (1998). The molluscicidal activity of crown of christ (*Euphorbia splendens* var. hislopii) latex on snails acting as intermediate hosts of *Schistosoma mansoni* and *Schistosoma haematobium. Am. J. Trop. Med. Hyg.*, 58(1): 7-10.

[68] Schall, V. T.; Vasconcellos M. C.; Rocha, R. S.; Souza, C. P.; Mendes, N. M. (2001). The control of the schistosome-transmitting snail *Biomphalaria glabrata* by the plant Molluscicide *Euphorbia splendens* var. *hislopii* (syn *milli* Des. Moul): a longitudinal field study in an endemic area in Brazil. *Acta Trop.*, 79: 165-170.

[69] Santos, AF; Azevedo, DP; Santos Mata, RC; Mendonça, DI; Sant'Ana, AE (2007). The lethality of *Euphorbia conspicua* to adults of *Biomphalaria glabrata*, cercaria of *Schistosoma mansoni* and larvae of *Artemia salina. Bioresour. Technol.*, 98(1): 135-139.

[70] Bezerra, DP; Militão, GC; Castro, FO; Pessoa, C; Moraes, MO; Silveira, ER; Lima, MA; Elmiro, FJ; Costa-Lotufo, LV (2007). Piplartine induces inhibition of leukemia cell proliferation triggering both apoptosis and necrosis pathways. *Toxicol. in Vitro*, 21(1): 1-8.

[71] Bezerra, DP; Castro, FO; Alves, AP; Pessoa, C; Moraes, MO; Silveira, ER; Lima, MA; Elmiro, FJ; Alencar, NM; Mesquita, RO; Lima, MW; Costa-Lotufo, LV (2008). In vitro and in vivo antitumor effect of 5-FU combined with piplartine and piperine. *J. Appl. Toxicol.*, 28(2): 156-163.

[72] Bodiwala, HS; Singh, G; Singh R; Dey, CS; Sharma, SS; Bhutani, KK; Singh, IP (2007). Antileishmanial amides and lignans from *Piper cubeba* and *Piper retrofractum. J. Nat. Med.,* 61(4): 418-421.

[73] Cotinguiba, F; Regasini, LO; Bolzani, VS; Debonsi, HM; Passerini, GD; Barretto, RM (2009). Piperamides and their derivatives as potential anti-trypanosomal agents. *Med. Chem. Res.*, 18(9): 703-711.

[74] Moraes, Jd; Nascimento, C; Lopes, PO; Nakano, E; Yamaguchi, LF; Kato, MJ; Kawano, T (2001). *Schistosoma mansoni*: in vitro schistosomicidal activity of piplartine. *Exp. Parasitol.*, 127 (2): 357-364.

[75] Blunt, JW; Copp, BR; Munro, MHG; Northcotec, PT; Prinsep, MR (2011) Marine natural products. *Nat. Prod. Rep.* 28: 196-268.

[76] Mayer, AMS; Rodríguez, AD; Berlinck, RGS; Fusetani, N (2011) Marine pharmacology in 2007-8: Marine compounds with antibacterial, anticoagulant, antifungal, anti-inflammatory, antimalarial, antiprotozoal, antituberculosis, and antiviral activities; affecting the immune and nervous system, and other miscellaneous mechanisms of action. *Comp. Biochem. Physiol. C Toxicol. Pharmacol.* 153: 191-222.

[77] Padilla, GM, Martin, DF (1973). Interactions of prymnesin with erythrocyte membranes. In: Martin DF, Padilla GM (eds) *Marine Pharmacognosy: Action of Marine Biotoxins at the Cellular Level.* Academic Press, New York, 265-295.

[78] Marchán, E; Arrieche, D; Henríquez, W; Crescente, O (2000). In vitro effect of an alkaloid isolated from *Amphimedon viridis* (Porifea) on promastigots of *Leishmania mexicana*. *Rev. Biol. Trop.*, 48Suppl 1:31-8.

[79] Reimão, JQ; Migotto, AE; Kossuga, MH; Berlinck, RGS; Tempone, AG (2008). Antiprotozoan activity of Brazilian marine cnidarian extracts and of a modified steroid from the octocoral *Carijoa riisei*. *Parasitol. Res.* 103: 1445–1450.

[80] Tempone, AG; Martins de Oliveira, C; Berlinck, RG (2011). Current approaches to discover marine antileishmanial natural products. *Planta Med.* 77(6): 572-85.

[81] Rand, GM; Wells, PG; McCarty, LS (1995). Introduction to Aquatic Toxicology. In: RAND, G. M. *Fundamentals of Aquatic Toxicology: Effects, Environmental Fate and Risk Assessment.* Washington, D. C., Taylor & Francis, 2 Ed, 3-67.

[82] Farré, M; Barceló, D (2003). Toxicity testing of wastewater and sewage sludge by biosensors, bioassays and chemical analysis. *Trends Analyt. Chem.*, 22(5): 299-310.

[83] Birge, WJ; Black, JA; Westerman, AG (1985). Short-term fish and amphibian tests for determining the effects of toxicant stress on early life stages and estimating chronic values for single compounds and complex effluents. *Environ. Toxicol. Chem.*, 49: 807-821.

[84] Mount, DIE; Norberg, TJ (1984). A seven day life cicle cladoceran toxicity test. *Environ. Toxicol. Chem.*, 3: 425-434.

[85] OECD (1992). *Guideline for Testing of Chemicals. Fish, Acute Toxicity* Test. 203, 12p.

[86] EPA, United States Environmental Protection Agency (2002). Short-term methods for estimating the chronic toxicity of effluents and receiving waters to freshwater organisms. U.S. *Environmental Protection Agency Office of Water,* 4th ed. Washington, DC, 1-40.

[87] OECD (2004). Guideline for Testing of Chemicals. *Daphnia* sp. Acute Immobilization Test. 202, 12p.

[88] OECD (2006). *Guideline for Testing of Chemicals. Freshwater Alga and Cyanobacteria*, Growth Inhibition Test. 201, 25p.

[89] EPA, United States Environmental Protection Agency (2012). *Ecological Effects Test Guidelines OCSPP 850.4500: Algal Toxicity,* 28p.

[90] Duncan, J (1985). The toxicology of plants molluscicides. *Pharmacology & Therapeutics,* v. 27, p. 243-264, 1985.

[91] Kawano T, Chaves WR, Simões LCG (1979) Effects of caffeine on embryonic development of *Biomphalaria glabrata. Cienc. Cult.* 31(11): 1266-1273.

[92] Arner J, Vila P, Plautz CZ (2009). Effects of Local Water Contaminants on the Development of Aquatic Organisms. *Sujur.* 1: 12-26.

In: Schistosomiasis
Editor: Adriana Erica Miele

ISBN: 978-1-63117-186-4

Chapter 5

Insights into Animal Schistosomiasis: From Surveillance to Control

Jose Ma. M. Angeles **[*]** ***and Shin-ichiro Kawazu***
National Research Center for Protozoan Diseases,
Obihiro University of Agriculture and Veterinary Medicine, Japan

Abstract

The role of animals in the transmission of schistosomiasis has not been given much importance, in fact massive efforts for the control of this disease have only been directed to humans. Other than human, more than 40 mammals are known to host the zoonotic *Schistosoma japonicum*. These animals somehow served as important "silent" sources of this parasitic disease in the transmission of the parasite and might be the loophole in the control of schistomiasis in endemic areas. However, minor steps toward animal schistosomiasis control have been taken, which include the use of recombinant antigens as a promising diagnostic tool for animals, as well as the admission of animals in the vaccination trials in China. This chapter will therefore tackle the importance of animals in the transmission of schistosomiasis, as well as the current

[*] Corresponding Author address: National Research Center for Protozoan Diseases, Obihiro University of Agriculture and Veterinary Medicine, Nishi 2-13, Inada-cho, Obihiro, Hokkaido 080-8555, Japan; E-mail: amoj28@gmail.com.

updates on the zoonotic surveillance and control of this parasitic disease. It also aims to promote the integration of the public health and veterinary sectors which might lead to the possible elimination of the zoonotic schistosomiasis.

Keywords: S*chistosoma japonicum*, zoonotic surveillance, veterinary schistosomiasis, diagnostic tools, vaccine

Zoonotic Schistosomiasis

The public health impact of animal schistosomiasis, such as the ones caused by *Schistosoma incognitum* among rodents [1], *S. currasoni* in sheeps [2], *S. hippopotami* and *S. edwardiense* found among hippopotamus [3] are very little compared to the zoonotic *S. japonicum. S. japonicum* is the major cause of zoonotic schistosomiasis in Asia, particularly in China, the Philippines and some parts of Indonesia. *S. japonicum* is known to infect over 40 different species of wild and domestic animals [4] belonging to the seven Orders in the Kingdom Mammalia (Figure 1).

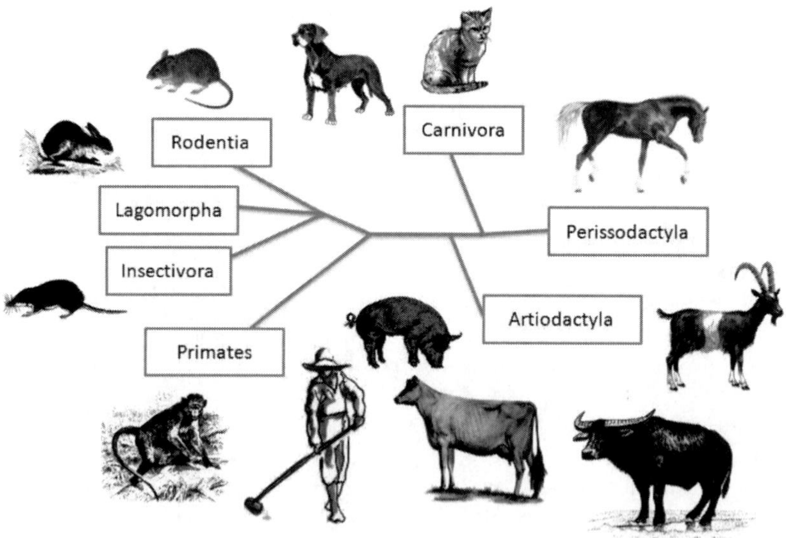

Figure 1. *Schistosoma japonicum* is known to infect a wide variety of animals belonging to different orders in the Kingdom Mammalia which includes human and other domesticated animals.

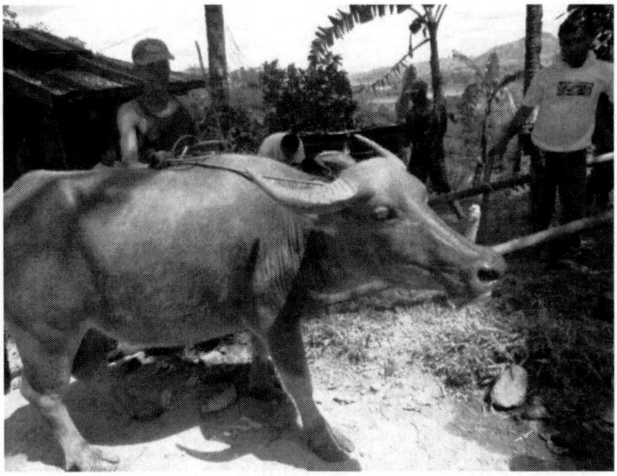

Figure 2. Domesticated animals including water buffaloes live so close to the human hosts that they even share infection caused by zoonotic parasites like *S. japonicum*.

These animals serve as reservoir hosts for the schistosome parasite which considerably complicates the control programs done in the endemic countries. These reservoir hosts play a significant role in maintaining the parasite, especially in areas where there is close co-existense between dense populations of humans and dense snail population. The close proximity of domesticated animals such as the dogs and water buffaloes to the human hosts as seen in Figure 2 is an important factor that can contribute in maintaining this parasite in endemic localities like the ones seen in rural agricultural areas. However, despite of this important role of animals in the parasite transmission, disease surveillance and control are only directed to the human hosts which might be a hindrance in obtaining the elusive disease elimination. On the other hand, the minor human schistosome *S. mekongi* was also found in animals such as dogs [5] and pigs [6]. Whether there is an active transmission between these animals and humans are not indicated so far with *S. mekongi*. The African *S. mansoni* is different with these two zoonotic schistosome species as the infected animals such as dogs most often do not shed the eggs in their excreta [7].

The Role of Animals in Schistosomiasis

Animals have already been implicated as possible sources of the schistosome parasite in schistosomiasis-endemic countries. In China, the most important reservoir hosts for *S. japonicum* are the bovines including the cattle and water buffalo [8-9]. Bovine defecation owned a large proportion of the environmental contamination for *S. japonicum* in China's schistosomiasis-endemic areas [10]. In Guanghui village, the relative transmission index (RTI) for schistosomiasis was calculated and found that water buffaloes were accounted for nearly 90% of the transmission, even higher than the 80.4% RTI from humans [11]. A study done using microsatellite markers has found that *S. japonicum* larval samples examined were divided into two clusters: one from the isolates from humans, cattle and water buffalo; and the other from dogs, cats, goats and pigs [12]. This suggested that transmission in China is more closely associated with bovines than the other domesticated animals.

In Indonesia, Izhar et al., have described that a small portion of domestic animals like water buffaloes and wild animals were found to be infected with the schistosome parasite [13]. On the other hand, a wide range of animals in the Philippines such as rats, cats, dogs, pigs, cattle and water buffaloes were found to be potential hosts for schistosomiasis using parasitological and immunological assays [14-16]. Furthermore, a population genetic study among these animal reservoir hosts, performed in one endemic province in the Philippines, suggests that there is a very high level of transmission between humans and dogs [17]. Water buffaloes, on the other hand, were examined in two separate studies and half of the examined population was found to be infected with *S. japonicum* [18-19]. These results strongly suggest that dogs and water buffaloes are the major reservoir hosts of schistosomiasis in the Philippines.

However, an important factor in the transmission of schistosomiasis is the number of schistosome eggs being passed in the excreta from the animal hosts that contaminates the environment, in addition to the duration of egg excretion and egg viability. Previous studies have shown that the number of eggs passed in the feces per female worm for each day differs between species [20]. Horses, goats and sheep shed the fewest, while the largest number of excreted eggs is seen in dogs and pigs as shown in Table 1. However, water buffaloes are more susceptible in acquiring *S. japonicum* than the other reservoir hosts as they spend more time in water, which might be contaminated with the infective *cercaria*. This water activity of the buffalo also largely contributes to the spread of the parasite making them important disease-transmitting hosts in the marshland areas of China. Furthermore, miracidial hatchability should be considered in assessing the actual contribution of the infected animals. It has been shown that excreted eggs from different host species have different hatching rates [21]. Therefore, it is more recommended to determine the number of miracidia per gram of stool rather than counting the number of eggs per gram of stool.

Table 1. Differences in the development of *Schistosoma japonicum* among domesticated animals [4]

Host	Worm establishment after one single infection (%)	No. of eggs shed in excreta per female worm per day	Persistence of egg excretion period post-infection
Dog	50-77	300-2000	8-12 months
Rabbit	37-75	100-500	1 year
Goat	39-76	50-100	1 year
Sheep	7-65	50-200	1 year
Pig	2-15	200-2000	6-10 months
Cow	41-65	150-600	>1 year
Water buffalo	5-16	150-600	6-8 months
Horse	<1	Few	1-4 months

Availability and abundance of the permissive hosts in an endemic area are also important in the transmission of the parasitosis. This makes the domesticated animals such as dogs, pigs and bovines to play a more significant role in the transmission than wild animals such as field rats, rabbits and monkeys. *S. japonicum* is also known to exist in Taiwan but the Formosan strain is zoophilic and cannot infect humans [22]. In early epidemiological studies done in Taiwan, domestic animals [23] including dogs, buffaloes, goats and pigs, as well as the wild *Rattus norvegicus*, *Crocidura murina*, *R. losea*, *Mus formosanus* and *R. rattus* [24] were found harboring the schistosome parasite. In 1986, an outbreak of schistosomiasis occurred at a cattle farm in Hanpao Fram, Fangyuan District, Chonghua County and have killed at least 15 cattle [25]. This indicates that this schistosome strain is a threat to the livestock animals not to humans.

Schistosome Infection in Animals

Unlike in the human host, the pathology caused by *S. japonicum* among the various animal reservoir hosts still remains to be cleared and is not much unraveled. Bovine schistosomiasis caused by *S. bovis* [26], *S. matthei* [27] and *S. spindale* [28] was known to show various lesions in the livers, intestinal tracts and other organs. On the other hand, canine schistosomiasis is mainly caused by the non-human schistosome *Heterobilharzia americana* in the North America which causes chronic intermittent dysentery, loss of weight, anemia and lymphadenopathy in dogs [29]. The pathological conditions seen with *S. japonicum* infection however differ among the reservoir host species.

In China, He et al., examined and compared the development rates of *S. japonicum* in mice, rats, guinea pigs, rabbits, goats, sheep, pigs, water buffalo, yellow cattle, horses and another 12 kinds of animal under identical conditions for up to 60 weeks [30]. The results presented that the development rates of the zoonotic schistosome in these hosts were quite different, with the highest infection rate of 60.3% seen in goats, 43.6% in yellow cattle, and 1% in water buffalo and horses. These differences in the parasite development inside the animal hosts are mainly due to the parasite clearance by the animal's immune system and non-immune system factors, called the self-cure phenomenon. The sharp drop in the worm burden after a period of *S. japonicum* infection was only seen in some animal hosts, such as rats, pigs [31] and water buffalo [32], but not in other susceptible animals like mice and yellow cattle.

Another study was done by Yang et al., comparing the development of *S. japonicum* in two important bovine hosts in China [33], namely the yellow cattle (*Bos taurus*) and water buffalo (*Bubalus bubalis*). The authors showed that the yellow cattle was found to be more suited to the development of *S. japonicum* than the water buffalo. Moreover, the cattle had more serious pathological damage. This high incidence of infection among the cattle might therefore possibly explain the significant mortality in this animal seen in most of the endemic areas. It was also shown that there is a decreased number of CD4+ T cells in yellow cattle, an increased proportion of CD8+ T cells in water buffalo, and a decreased CD4/CD8 ratios in both species after schistosome challenge, suggesting that CD4+ T cells could be an integral component in the immune response against the parasite and might explain the worm development in yellow cattle. Results of an earlier study on the schistosome-sensitive mice were consistent with the above reported observations [34]. Yang et al., also compared the general morphology and ultrastructure of adult schistosomes derived from the two bovine hosts as well their gene expression profiles using high-throughput microarray technology [35]. Results of the ultrastructure observations showed that the schistosomes from water buffalo differ from those of the yellow cattle as the adult worms have a collapsed and loose surface, with fewer spines and sensory papillae, dissolved cytoplasmic organelles and more vacuole structures in the male worm tegument. On the other hand, their results also identified genes that were differentially expressed in worms from the two natural hosts. Schistosomes extracted from water buffalo overexpressed genes associated with the stimulus response, and lipid and nucleotide metabolism, and protein kinase and phosphatase; genes associated with reproduction, anatomical structure morphogenesis and multifunctional motif were underexpressed. These differentially expressed genes (mainly involved in nucleotide, energy and lipid metabolisms, transcription, transport and signaling pathways) greatly affect the survival and development of schistosomes in different natural host species. These results provide significant information that will possibly help in understanding the differences in the developmental rates among different reservoir hosts as well as the serious pathological damage seen in some animals. Further elaboration of the mechanism of this self-cure phenomenon might also be important in the development of schistosome vaccine.

Field rats, on the other hand, were also known to have high percentages of infection in extensive field surveys done in China, the Philippines and Indonesia [36-37]. Rodents were seen to have the highest infection prevalence in hill areas within Anhui Province of China whereas the cattle had the highest infection prevalence in the marshlands [38]. However, the risk of transmission from these rodents seems to be minimal as the schistosome worms were found to be trapped in the lungs and only rarely mature to produce eggs [39]. This suggested that although the rodents are infected with the parasites, the importance of these animals in the disease transmission is definitive low. In contrast to this, epidemiological studies done in endemic areas in China and the Philippines showed excretion of many viable eggs in the feces from field rats [39-40]. Although field rats at individual level might not contribute significantly to transmission, the presence of enormous number of field rats in endemic areas might pose a potential problem for the spread of the parasite.

As shown in Table 1, worm establishment is generally low in pigs. There are also no visible clinical signs among the infected pigs except from the diarrhea at the onset of patency [41-42]. Due to acquired immunity and short life span, the role of the pigs in the disease transmission is somehow negligible. However, sows infected at 10 weeks of gestation showed transplacental infection [43]. This proved that pigs can still be a threat in transmitting the disease in endemic areas where pig-raising is usually done.

Animal Surveillance

Detection of the schistosome eggs in the stool samples through microscopy is still the gold standard for schistosomiasis diagnosis in both humans and animals. Stool microscopy is known to show low sensitivity in diagnosing low infection and in areas with low endemicity. Therefore, more accurate coprological techniques were developed for schistosomiasis diagnosis such as the Danish Bilharziasis Laboratory (DBL) technique [44] and the formalin-ethyl acetate sedimentation-digestion (FEA-SD) technique. Carabin et al., measured and compared the specificity and sensitivity of the filtration and sedimentation DBL using one, two, three, four or five consecutive days of stool samples from various animal hosts in the Philippines [14]. Results of this study showed that the DBL technique has at least 96% sensitivity when three stool samples or more are collected on three separate days and at least 91% specificity when three stool samples or less were collected on three separate days. This therefore suggested that the maximum sensitivity and specificity DBL can achieve is by collecting three stool samples on separate days and results based on only one stool sample underestimate the true prevalence of animal infection.

On the other hand, FEA-SD has shown to have improved visualization of *S. japonicum* eggs in bovine feces [45]. This technique includes filtration, sedimentation, potassium hydroxide digestion and centrifugation steps prior to microscopy discriminating nearly 70% of debris from the fecal samples and rendering the remaining debris translucent. This will be useful in rural endemic localities as it is not costly and does not require expensive equipments.

As a better alternative for the less sensitive coprological methods, crude antigen-based immunodiagnostic techniques like circum-oval precipitin test (COPT) and enzyme-linked immunosorbent assay (SEA-ELISA, SWAP-ELISA) might be preferably used. However, crude antigens are known to cause cross-reactions with other helminthiasis, affecting its specificity. In addition, massive production of crude egg antigen for large scale diagnostic purposes such as epidemiological surveys is somewhat difficult and tedious. To possibly replace the crude antigens, recombinant antigens which are easier to produce have been characterized and studied for their diagnostic potentials. Only a few defined antigens have been identified so far for serological diagnosis of animal schistosomiasis (see Table 2). These antigens, which are tested using animal samples, yielded remarkable sensitivity and specificity with a range of 78 to 100%. These recombinant antigens therefore can be used in improving the schistosomiasis surveillance in endemic areas.

However, the success of zoonotic surveillance cannot rely on sensitivity and specificity. The universality of the antigens for schistosomiasis diagnosis is another criterion that needs to be considered.

Table 2. List of promising recombinant *S. japonicum* antigens characterized and tested for the diagnosis of animal schistosomiasis

Antigen	Species
26 kDa Glutathione-S-transferase (Sjc26GST)	Water Buffalo [46]
Fructose-1,6-biphosphate aldolase (FBPA)	Water Buffalo [47]
Gynecophoral canal protein (GCP), tetraspanin fragment (Sj23) and 28 kDa GST (rSjGCP-Sj23-Sj28)	Cattle [48]
Thioredoxin peroxidase-1 (SjTPx1)	Cattle [48], human [49], water buffalo [18]
Elongation factor 1-alpha (rSjEF1)	Cattle [48]
Large hydrophilic domain of Sj23 (LHD-Sj23)	Cattle [50]
Dentin sialophosphoprotein (Sj1TR)	Human [49], water buffalo [18]

The majority of these antigens were examined in either the cattle or water buffalo. Tandem repeat protein Sj1TR was tested for both humans [49] and water buffaloes [18] but results showed that it was only good for diagnosing the latter. Among the antigens tested, only thioredoxin peroxidase-1 (SjTPx-1) showed a promising diagnostic capability as it was shown to have remarkable diagnostic potentials in a number of species which includes human [49], cattle [48], water buffalo [18] and dog (Angeles et al., unpublished data) serum samples. Examining the potential of SjTPx-1 on other animal reservoir hosts like pigs and rats to develop a more universal diagnostic test for both human and animals is now underway. A multi-species diagnostic test will surely strengthen the disease surveillance for schistosomiasis, ensuring the detection of all active transmission mechanisms involved in one endemic area.

In the case of epidemiological studies and surveillance of animal infection in areas that have reached elimination level, a more sensitive and specific diagnostic test is highly required. Molecular techniques like polymerase chain reaction (PCR) have been developed for detecting animal infection. Wu et al. have compared stool microscopy with a real-time PCR detection of *S. japonicum* mitochondrial DNA in water buffalo stool samples [19]. Their results showed a very big difference in prevalence between the two techniques and suggested that microscopic-based techniques dramatically underestimate the prevalence of *S. japonicum* infection among the water buffaloes. Therefore there is really a need for better and improved diagnostic techniques to reach the real picture of animal transmission for schistosomiasis.

Schistosomiasis Control in Animals

Control measures done in schistosomiasis-endemic countries consist mainly of community-based praziquantel chemotherapy, sanitation, supply of safe water, provision of personal protection, snail elimination and health education.. However, schistosomiasis control is complicated such that these parasites are so thoroughly integrated into the ecosystems, in which they occur, making the control at the community level very difficult, despite available control mechanisms. In Japan, *S. japonicum* was eliminated in 1977 just before the drug praziquantel became available [51]. This success story was largely based on ecological approaches strongly implemented by the Japanese government. In contrast, most underdeveloped countries have neither the political will nor the infrastructure, nor enough funding for the control measures leading to the steady existence of schistosomiasis until this very day.

Despite over 50 years of concerted efforts for its control, schistosomiasis still remains to be a major public health concern in China [52]. Transmission interruption had reached 60% and transmission control 14.5% of all the schistosome-endemic areas in China, until the mid-80's. Ecological factors like flooding, however, led to snail diffusion and re-emergence of schistosomiasis in the Yangtze River in recent years [53].

In the Philippines, chemotherapy has made the prevalence and morbidity of schistosomiasis dropping significantly in many areas. [54]. But in the past few years, emergence of two new endemic foci has been reported primarily due to the mobility of the people and other ecological factors [55]. New effective control strategies against schistosomiasis therefore should be studied and applied to eradicate this disease of antiquity.

Inclusion of zoonotic interventions in the national control programs done in these endemic countries is a much-needed strategy. Previous studies have shown that animal interventions can successfully cause decline in the prevalence of *S. japonicum* infection among humans [56-57]. In a five-year praziquantel-based intervention study done around the Poyang Lake in Jiangxi Province, China, simultaneous treatment of the bovine hosts has proven to be effective in the reduction of human schistosomiasis cases. This has significantly changed the epidemiological situation in China, such that they now consider schistosomiasis primarily as a bovine disease that can be transmitted to humans and, therefore, bovine schistosomiasis should be managed first before the human one.

Rapid re-infection is indeed possible for schistosomiasis. This requires repeated treatments, which raise concerns on the development of drug resistance. Resistance for the anti-schistosome drug praziquantel has only been reported for *S. mansoni* in Africa [58-62], but not yet for the zoonotic *S. japonicum*. Seto et al. measured the efficacy of praziquantel for the treatment of *S. japonicum* in humans by conducting a cross-sectional survey in 33 villages of Sichuan Province and concluded that praziquantel remains to be an effective drug for treating this parasitosis [63]. Nevertheless, other strategies should be done to complement existing control measures and therefore, development of a protective vaccine against human and animal schistosomiasis might be an essential component on the long-term disease control. In addition, on one hand zoonotic transmission made the control programs more complex, on the other it also provides opportunities for novel approaches in vaccine development to prevent the human disease.

Development of transmission-blocking veterinary vaccines that can be used for livestock animals is a complementary approach in schistosomiasis control. Radiation-attenuated cercarial vaccines have been successfully tested in water buffaloes [64] and pigs [65] under field conditions in China. However, many inherent problems were found using the cercarial vaccines, such as difficulty on producing quality-controlled, reproducible batches of these vaccines. Thus, vaccine researches resorted to the use of either the protein or DNA vaccines that might be effective [66-69]. Table 3 shows the list of the *S. japonicum* protein and DNA vaccines tested in domesticated animal reservoir hosts.

The protective efficacy of the schistosome-derived glutathione S-transferase (GST) family has been thoroughly investigated. The schistosome GST enzymes, which exist as 26- (Sj26GST) and 28-kDa (Sj28GST) molecules, have demonstrated remarkable effects on the fecundity of the adult parasites. Vaccination of sheep with native unfractionated *S. japonicum* GSTs has induced 53% partial protection [76]. Recombinant Sj26GST (reSj26GST) is capable of stimulating anti-fecundity immunity in pigs [79], water buffaloes [77] and sheep [75] with more than 50% egg reduction. Wu et al. demonstrated that vaccination of cattle with reSj26GST could elicit protection for at least 12 months and a 30% worm burden reduction [78]. Natural field challenge of recombinant Sj28GST (reSj28GST) has shown 33% worm reduction and 36% fecal egg reduction in water buffaloes, but not in cattle [80]. In sheep reSj28GST has induced 34-69% worm reduction, 56-69% liver egg reduction and 43-60% fecal egg reduction [75].

Cytosolic fatty acid-binding protein or SjFABPc is a molecule known to be crucial for egg production [88] and therefore, has been suggested as a valuable vaccine candidate or drug target for lowering the pathology of the infection through reduction or abrogation of egg production. Liu et al. have shown that this molecule might be a promising vaccine antigen by providing protective efficacies in both rats and sheep without adjuvants [81].

Table 3. List of *S. japonicum* protein and DNA vaccines tested in domesticated animals

Antigen	Animal Tested
Protein vaccine	
Paramyosin (Sj97)	*Native*: sheep [70] *Recombinant*: water buffalo [71], pig [72]
Integral membrane protein (Sj23)	*Native*: water buffalo [73] *Recombinant*: Water buffalo [73], cattle [74], sheep [75]
26-kDA GST (Sj26GST)	*Native*: sheep [76] *Recombinant:* water buffalo [77], cattle [78], pig [79], sheep [75]
28-kDa GST (Sj28GST)	*Recombinant*: sheep [75], water buffalo [80] , cattle [80]
FABP (Sj14)	*Recombinant*: sheep [81]
DNA Vaccines	
Triose-phosphate isomerase (SjTPI)	Pig [82], water buffalo [83,84]
Integral membrane protein (Sj23)	Pig [85], sheep [73], water buffalo [73,83], cattle [86]
28-kDa GST (Sj28GST)	Water buffalo [86], cattle [86]
31/32-kDa protein (Sj31/32)	Goat [87]

The muscle protein paramyosin, as well, has shown 42 to 48.8% liver egg reduction in water buffaloes [71] and 32.9 to 34.5% worm burden reduction in pigs [72].

All in all, the use of protein vaccines resorted to a worm burden reduction ranging from 17 to 60% in these animals. On the other hand, DNA vaccines lead to a smaller reduction of worm burden (16-65%) and liver egg burden (19-72%). The tetraspanin integral membrane protein (Sj23) was initially shown to induce protection was a synthetic peptide vaccine [73-75] and then, as a plasmid DNA vaccine . This latter shows protective efficacy in mice, sheeps, pigs and water buffaloes. Shi et al. showed that vaccination using Sj23 plasmid DNA has led to significant adult worm reductions in sheep and water buffaloes [73]. Sj23 plasmid DNA vaccine was also shown to partially protect cattle naturally exposed to the parasite over several months [74].

The glycolytic pathway enzyme triose-phosphate isomerase (TPI) has long been targeted as schistosomiasis vaccine candidate for *S. mansoni*. For *S. japonicum*, Zhu et al. determined its efficacy in naïve pigs by vaccination with the TPI DNA plasmid (SjCTPI) alone or in conjunction with IL-12 plasmids [84]. SjCTPI vaccine showed a more pronounced effect on reducing female worm burdens (53.6-59.6%). In addition, SjCTPI has reduced liver egg numbers (49.4%) which was significantly enhanced by the addition of IL-12 (65.8%). Protective immunity was also seen in experimental *S. japonicum* infected water buffaloes followed by co-immunization of SjCTPI DNA plasmid fused with heat shock protein 70 and IL-12 DNA [85].

Sj31 and Sj32 are two *S. japonicum* vaccine candidate antigens, which were particularly promising to induce protective immunity in mice [89-90]. Tang et al. produced the DNA vaccine formulations of the two antigens, which were used to immunize goats [87]. Results of their experiment showed a strong anamnestic antibody response with significant reduction in worm burden (20.9-31.6%).

Although these results are somehow encouraging, further extensive experimental and field-based natural challenge trials are still needed to determine whether these animal vaccines will really reduce transmissions in schistosomiasis. Finally, field trials, including the measurement of the effect of some of these animal vaccines in the prevalence of human schistosomiasis are presently under study in China.

Aside from the vaccine development, the Chinese government has replaced the bovines with machines across the endemic agricultural areas for schistosomiasis control [91]. The new intervention which includes the provision of mechanized farm equipment and removes the cattle from snail-infested grasslands also aims to improve sanitation by supplying tap water and building lavatories and latrines, providing boats with fecal-matter containers and implementing an intensive health education program. In the assessment done after three transmission seasons, the rate of human infection has decreased to less than 1% in intervention areas. This proved that the role of the bovine animals in the transmission of the parasite has greatly reduced. However, this control strategy might promote the possibility of making the rodents a major reservoir host in currently bovine-maintained transmission sites. Therefore, rodent surveillance should also be in place in the event that such outcome occurred to safeguard the current achieved reduction in human disease prevalence.

Integration of Veterinary and Medical Sectors

It has been historically known that joint efforts of both veterinary and medical sectors are needed to control zoonotic diseases. All throughout history, veterinary medicine has played a significant role in public health and has been tapped in many globally-significant medical circumstances involving zoonoses, such as outbreaks of avian influenza and control of rabies. Zoonoses, which represent up to 75% of the emerging pathogens [92], have a major impact on human health in the developing world. However, due to the low level of immediate attention these diseases have elicited, most of the zoonotic diseases affecting men, like schistosomiasis, are neglected and do not include the required veterinary control measures. Schistosomiasis has been known since the time of the pharaohs in Egypt but until now, its elimination has been a steady challenge for the endemic countries.

Therefore there is a call for the integration of public health and veterinary sectors in the fight against schistosomiasis, and this can be done via the 'One Health' strategy [93]. This concept is a worldwide strategy in controlling zoonoses by expanding interdisciplinary collaborations and communications in all aspects of healthcare for humans, animals and the environment. The goal of this strategy is to advance health care by accelerating biomedical research discoveries, enhancing public health efficacy, expeditiously expanding the scientific knowledge base, and improving medical education and clinical care.

Current advances in *Schistosoma* research programs, like the completion of the genome project, make way for strategizing new disease elimination programs. However, having a synergistic effort from both the medical and veterinary health sectors is the real challenge that needs to be urgently addressed for the future of this ancient parasitic disease.

References

[1] Bunnag T, Thirachandra S, Impand P, Vorasanta P, Imlarp S (1983). *Schistosoma incognitum* and its zoonotic potential role in Phitsanulok and Phichit provinces, northern Thailand. *Southeast Asian J. Trop. Med. Public Health* 14(2): 163-170.

[2] Vercruysse J, Rollinson D, van Heerden M, Southgate VR (2003). On the longevity of *Schistosoma curassoni*. *J. Helminthol.* 77(1): 89-90.

[3] Morgan JA, DeJong RJ, Kazibwe F, Mkoji GM, Loker ES (2003). A newly-identified lineage of *Schistosoma*. *Int. J. Parasitol.* 33(9): 977-985.

[4] He YX, Salafsky B, Ramaswamy K (2001). Host-parasite relationships of *Schistosoma japonicum* in mammalian hosts. *Trends Parasitol.* 7: 320-324.

[5] Matsumoto J, Muth S, Socheat D, Matsuda H (2002). The first reported cases of canine schistosomiasis mekongi in Cambodia. *Southeast Asian J. Trop. Med. Public Health* 33(3): 458-461.

[6] Strandgaard H, Johansen MV, Pholsena K, Teixayavong, Christensen NO (2001). The pig as a host for *Schistosoma mekongi* in Laos. *J. Parasitol.* 87(3): 708-709.

[7] Muller R (2000). Dogs zoonoses and public health. In: Macpherson CNL Meslin FX &Wandeler AI, ed. CABI Publishing: NY USA, 150-151.

[8] Gray DJ, Williams GM, Li Y, Chen H, Forsyth SJ, Li RS, Barnett AG, Guo J, Ross AG, Feng Z, McManus DP (2009). A cluster-randomized intervention trial against *Schistosoma japonicum* in the People's Republic of China: bovine and human transmission. *PLoS One* 4: e5900.

[9] Shi F, Zhang Y, Lin J, Zuo X, Shen W, Cai Y, Ye P, Bickle QD, Taylor MG (2002). Field testing of *Schistosoma japonicum* DNA vaccines in cattle in China. *Vaccine* 20: 3629-3631.

[10] Zheng J, Zheng QS, Wang XF, Hua ZH (1997). Influence of livestock husbandry on schistosomiasis transmission in mountainous regions of Yunnan province. *SE Asian J. Trop. Med. Public Health* 28: 291-295.

[11] Wang TP, Vang Johansen M, Zhang SQ, Wang FF, Wu WD, Zhang GH, Pan XP, Ju Y, Ørnbjerg N (2005). Transmission of *Schistosoma japonicum* by humans and domestic animals in the Yangtze River valley, Anhui province, China. *Acta Trop.* 96(2-3): 198-204.

[12] Wang TP, Shrivastava J, Johansen MV, Zhang SQ, Wang FF Webster JP (2006). Does multiple hosts mean multiple parasites? Population genetic structure of *Schistosoma japonicum* between definitive host species. *Int. J. Parasitol.* 36(12): 1317-1325.

[13] Izhar A, Sinaga RM, Sudomo M, Wardiyo ND (2002). Recent situation of schistosomiasis in Indonesia. *Acta Trop.* 82: 283-288.

[14] Carabin H, Balolong E, Joseph L, McGarvey ST, Johansen MV, Fernandez T, Willingham AL, Olveda R (2005). Estimating sensitivity and specificity of a faecal examination for *Schistosoma japonicum* infection in cats, dogs, water buffaloes, pigs, and rats in Western Samar

and Sorsogon Provinces, The Philippines. *Int. J. Parasitol.* 35: 1517-1524.

[15] Fernandez TJ Jr, Tarafder MR, Balolong E Jr, Joseph L, Willingham AL 3rd, Bélisle P, Webster JP, Olveda RM, McGarvey ST, Carabin H (2007). Prevalence of *Schistosoma japonicum* infection among animals in fifty villages of Samar province, the Philippines. *Vector Borne Zoonotic Dis.* 7: 147-155.

[16] Matsumoto J, Kirinoki M, Kawai S, Chigusa Y, Ilagan EJ, Ducusin BE, Yasuraoka K, Matsuda H (1999). Prevalence of schistosomiasis japonica among schoolchildren and animal reservoirs in Oriental Mindoro, Philippines. *Jpn J. Trop. Med. Hyg.* 27: 175-180.

[17] Rudge JW, Carabin H, Balolong E, Tallo V, Shrivastava J, Lu DB, Basanez MG, Olveda R, McGarvey ST, Webster JP (2008). Population genetics of *Schistosoma japonicum* within the Philippines suggest high levels of transmission between humans and dogs. *PLoS Negl. Trop. Dis.* 2(11): e340.

[18] Angeles JM, Goto Y, Kirinoki M, Asada M, Leonardo L, Tongol-Rivera P, Villacorte E, Inoue N, Chigusa Y, Kawazu S (2012). Utilization of ELISA using thioredoxin peroxidase-1 and tandem repeat proteins for diagnosis of *Schistosoma japonicum* infection among water buffaloes. *PLoS Negl. Trop. Dis.* 6(8): e1800.

[19] Wu HW, Qin YF, Chu K, Meng R, Liu Y, McGarvey ST, Olveda R, Acosta L, Ji MJ, Fernandez T, Friedman JF, Kurtis JD, 2010. High prevalence of *Schistosoma japonicum* infection in water buffaloes in the Philippines assessed by real-time polymerase chain reaction. *Am. J. Trop. Med. Hyg* 82: 646-652.

[20] Ho YH, He YX, 1963. On the host specificity of *Schistosoma japonicum*. *Chin Med J* 82: 403-414.

[21] Li YF, Xu ZY, Leng JL, Dong MH, Zhu Q, He SY (1991). Experimental study on egg hatching rate of schistosomiasis japonica. *Chin. J. Schisto Contr.* 3: 33-35.

[22] Hsu HF, Hsu Li SY (1956). On the infectivity of the Formosan strain of *Schistosoma japonicum* in *Homo sapiens*. *Am. J. Trop. Med. Hyg.* 5: 521-528.

[23] Hsu HF, Hsu Li SY, Chu KY (1954). Schistosomiasis japonica among domestic animals in Formosa. *Riv. Parasitol.* 15: 461.

[24] Hsu HF, Hsu Li SY (1955). Studies on schistosomiasis japonica in Formosa IV. Wild rats and other small mammals as reservoir host of *Schistosoma japonicum* in Formosa. *Ann. Acad. Sin.* 2: 147.

[25] Wang JS, Tung KC, Chang JP (1988). Studies on the bovine schistosomiasis 1986 on Taiwan: pathological and scanning electron microscope observations. *Proceedings of the Sino-Japanese Symposium on Parasitic Zoonoses* 39-44.

[26] Hussein MF, Tartour G, Imbabi SE, Ali KE (1975). The pathology of naturally-occurring bovine schistosomiasis in the Sudan. *Ann. Trop. Med. Parasitol.* 69(2): 217-25.

[27] Lawrence JA (1978). The pathology of *Schistosoma mattheei* infection in the ox 1. Lesions attributable to the eggs. *J. Comp. Pathol.* 88(1): 1-14.

[28] Fransen J, De Bont J, Vercruysse J, Van Aken D, Southgate VR, Rollinson D (1990). Pathology of natural infections of *Schistosoma spindale* Montgomery, 1906, in cattle. *J. Comp. Pathol.* 103(4): 447-455.

[29] Johnson E (2010). Canine schistosomiasis in North America: an underdiagnosed disease with an expanding distribution. *Compend. Contin. Educ. Vet.* 32(3): E1-4.

[30] He YX, Yang HZ, Mao SB (1960). Host specificity of schistosomiasis japonica I: The developmental rates, distribution and survival in mammals. *Chin. Med. J.* 46: 470-475.

[31] Lu MY Li YF, Lin DD (2010). The self-cure phenomenon in buffalo and pig infected with *Schistosoma japonicum* and its mechanism. *Int. J. Med. Parasit Dis.* 37(3): 184-188.

[32] Luo XF, Lin SY, Lin ZY, Zhang CF, Wu WR (1988). Observation of the self-cure phenomenon of water buffalo infection with *Schistosoma japonicum*. *Chin. J. Vet. Sci. Technol* 8: 42-44.

[33] Yang J, Fu Z, Feng X, Shi Y, Yuan C, Liu J, Hong Y, Li H, Lu K, Lin J (2012). Comparison of worm development and host immune responses in natural hosts of *Schistosoma japonicum*, yellow cattle and water buffalo. *BMC Vet. Res.* 8: 25.

[34] Kalinkovich A, Weisman Z, Greenberg Z, Nahmias J, Eitan S, Stein M, Bentwich RZ (1998): Decreased CD4 and increased CD8 counts with T cell activation is associated with chronic helminth infection. *Clin. Exp. Immunol.* 114(3): 414-421.

[35] Yang J, Feng X, Fu Z, Yuan C, Hong Y, Shi Y, Zhang M, Liu J, Li H, Lu K, Lin J (2012). Ultrastructural observation and gene expression profiling of *Schistosoma japonicum* derived from two natural reservoir hosts, water buffalo and yellow cattle. *PLoS One* 7(10): e47660.

[36] Mitchell GF, Garcia EG, Wood SM, Diasanta R, Almonte R, Calica E, Davern KM, Tiu WU (1990). Studies on the sex ratio of worms in schistosome infections. *Parasitology* 101(1): 27-34.

[37] Fedorko JM (1999). *Schistosoma japonicum* in the black rat, *Rattus rattus mindanensis*, from Leyte, Philippines in relation to *Oncomelania* snail colonies with reference to other endoparasites. *Southeast Asian J. Trop. Med. Public Health* 30(2): 343-9.

[38] Lu DB, Wang TP, Rudge JW, Donnelly CA, Fang GR, Webster JP (2010). Contrasting reservoirs for *Schistosoma japonicum* between marshland and hilly regions in Anhui, China--a two-year longitudinal parasitological survey. *Parasitology* 137(1): 99-110.

[39] Wu K (1957). Schistosomiasis japonica among domestic and wild animals in China. *Chin. Vet. J.* 3: 98-100.

[40] Dumag PU, Gajudo CE, Sena CY, Cardenas EC, Fementira EB (1981). Epidemiology of animal schistosomiasis in the Philippines. *Philippine J. Anim. Ind.* 36: 1-23.

[41] Hurst MH, Willingham AL 3rd, Lindberg R (2000). Tissue responses in experimental schistosomiasis japonica in the pig: a histopathologic study of different stages of single low- or high-dose infections. *Am. J. Trop. Med. Hyg* 62(1): 45-56.

[42] Yason CV and Novilla MN (1984). Clinical and pathologic features of experimental *Schistosoma japonicum* infection in pigs. *Vet. Parasitol.* 17: 47-64.

[43] Willingham AL 3rd, Johansen MV, Bøgh HO, Ito A, Andreassen J, Lindberg R, Christensen NO, Nansen P (1999). Congenital transmission of *Schistosoma japonicum* in pigs. *Am. J. Trop. Med. Hyg* 60(2): 311-312.

[44] Willingham AL, Johansen MJ, Barnes EH (1998). A new technique for counting *Schistosoma japonicum* eggs in pig faeces. *Southeast Asian J. Trop. Med. Public Health* 29: 128-130.

[45] Xu B, Gordon CA, Hu W, McManus DP, Chen HG, Gray DJ, Ju C, Zeng XJ, Gobert GN, Ge J, Lan WM, Xie SY, Jiang WS, Feng Z (2012). A novel procedure for precise quantification of *Schistosoma japonicum* eggs in bovine feces. *PLoS Negl. Trop. Dis.* 6(11): e1885.

[46] Cheng PC, Tsaihong JC, Lee KM (2007). Application of recombinant Sjc26GST for serodiagnosis of *Schistosoma japonicum* infection in water buffalo (*Bos buffelus*). *Vet. Parasitol.* 150: 314-320.

[47] Peng SY, Lee KM, Tsaihong JC, Cheng PC, Fan PC (2008). Evaluation of recombinant fructose-1,6-biphosphate aldolase ELISA test for the

diagnosis of *Schistosoma japonicum* in water buffaloes. *Res. Vet. Science* 85: 527-533.

[48] Jin YM, Lu K, Zhou WF, Fu ZQ, Liu JM, Shi YJ, Li H, Lin JJ (2010). Comparison of recombinant proteins from *Schistosoma japonicum* for schistosomiasis diagnosis. *Clin. Vaccine Immuno.* 17: 476-480.

[49] Angeles JM, Goto Y, Kirinoki M, Leonardo LR, Tongol-Rivera P, P, Villacorte E, Inoue N, Chigusa Y, Kawazu S (2011). Human antibody response to thioredoxin peroxidase-1 and tandem repeat proteins as immunodiagnostic antigen candidates for Schistosoma japonicum infection. *Am. J. Trop. Med. Hyg* 85: 674-679.

[50] Li Y, Wang L, Fang R, Nie H, Zhou Y, Zhao J, Hua M (2012). Establishment and evaluation of an iELISA using the recombinant membrane protein LHD-Sj23 for the serodiagnosis of *Schistosoma japonicum* infection in cattle in China. *Vet. Parasitol.* 188: 247-254.

[51] Minai M, Hosaka Y, Ohta N (2003). Historical view of schistosomiasis japonica in Japan: implementation and evaluation of disease-control strategies in Yamanashi Prefecture. *Parasitol. Int.* 52: 321-326.

[52] Zhou XN, Wang LY, Chena MG, Wua XH, Jiang QW, Chen XY, Zheng J, Utzinger J (2005). The public health significance and control of schistosomiasis in China—then and now. *Acta Trop.* 96: 97-105.

[53] Zhou XN, Lin DD, Yang HM, Chen HG, Sun LP, Yang GJ, Hong QB, Brown L, Malone JB (2002). Use of Landsat TM satellite surveillance data to measure the impact of the 1998 flood on snail intermediate host dispersal in the lower Yangtze River basin. *Acta Trop* 82: 199-205.

[54] Leonardo LR, Acosta LP, Olveda RM, Aligui GDL (2002). Difficulties and strategies in the control of schistosomiasis in the Philippines. *Acta Trop* 82: 295-299.

[55] Leonardo L, Rivera P, Saniel O, Antonio Solon J, Chigusa Y, Villacorte E, Christoper Chua J, Moendeg K, Manalo D, Crisostomo B, Sunico L, Boldero N, Payne L, Hernandez L, Velayudhan R (2013). New endemic foci of schistosomiasis infections in the Philippines. *Acta Trop.*, 10.1016/j.actatropica.2013.03.015 [ePub ahed of print].

[56] Gray DJ, Williams GM, Li Y, Chen H, Forsyth SJ, Li RS, Barnett AG, Guo J, Ross AG, Feng Z, McManus DP (2009). A cluster-randomized intervention trial against *Schistosoma japonicum* in the People's Republic of China: bovine and human transmission. *PLoS One* 4: e5900.

[57] Guo J, Li Y, Gray D, Ning A, Hu G, Chen H, Davis GM, Sleigh AC, Feng Z, McManus DP, Williams GM (2006). A drug-based intervention study on the importance of buffaloes for human *Schistosoma japonicum*

infection around Poyang Lake, People's Republic of China. *Am. J. Trop. Med. Hyg*. 74: 335-341.

[58] Ismail M, Metwally A, Farghaly A, Bruce J, Tao LF, Bennett JL (1996). Characterization of isolates of *Schistosoma mansoni* from Egyptian villagers that tolerate high doses of praziquantel. *Am. J. Trop. Med. Hyg*. 55: 214-218.

[59] Ismail M, Botros S, Metwally A, William S, Farghally A, Tao LF, Day TA, Bennett JL (1999). Resistance to praziquantel: direct evidence from *Schistosoma mansoni* isolated from Egyptian villagers. *Am. J. Trop. Med. Hyg*. 60: 932-935.

[60] Gryseels B, Stelma FF, Talla I, van Dam GJ, Polman K, Sow S, Diaw M, Sturrock RF, Doehring-Schwerdtfeger E, Kardorff R (1994). Epidemiology, immunology and chemotherapy of *Schistosoma mansoni* infections in a recently exposed community in Senegal. *Trop. Geogr. Med*. 46: 209-219.

[61] Stelma FF, Sall S, Daff B, Sow S, Niang M, Gryseels B (1997). Oxamniquine cures *Schistosoma mansoni* infection in a focus in which cure rates with praziquantel are unusually low. *J. Infect Dis*. 176: 304-307.

[62] Gryseels B, Mbaye A, De Vlas SJ, Stelma FF, Guissé F, Van Lieshout L, Faye D, Diop M, Ly A, Tchuem-Tchuenté LA, Engels D, Polman K (2001). Are poor responses to praziquantel for the treatment of *Schistosoma mansoni* infections in Senegal due to resistance? An overview of the evidence. *Trop. Med. Int. Health* 6: 864-873.

[63] Seto EYW, Wong BK, Lu D, Zhong B (2011). Human schistosomiasis resistance to praziquantel in China: should we be worried? *Am. J. Trop. Med. Hyg*. 85(1): 74-82.

[64] Shi YE, Jiang CF, Han JJ, Li YL, Ruppel A (1990). *Schistosoma japonicum*: an ultraviolet-attenuated cercarial vaccine applicable in the field for water buffaloes. *Exp. Parasitol*. 71(1): 100-106.

[65] Shi YE, Jiang CF, Han JJ, Li YL, Ruppel A (1993). Immunization of pigs against infection with *Schistosoma japonicum* using ultraviolet-attenuated cercariae. *Parasitology* 106: 459-462.

[66] McManus DP (2000). A vaccine against Asian schistosomiasis: the story unfolds. *Int. J. Parasitol*. 30: 265-271.

[67] McManus DP, Bartley PB (2004). A vaccine against Asian schistosmiasis. *Parasitol. Int*. 53: 163-173.

[68] McManus DP, Loukas A (2008). Current status of vaccines for schistosomiasis. *Clin. Microbiol. Rev*. 21(1): 225-242.

[69] Wu ZD, Lu ZY, Yu XB (2005). Development of a vaccine against *Schistosoma japonicum* in China: a review. *Acta Trop.* 96: 106-116.

[70] Taylor MG, Huggins MC, Shi F, Lin J, Tian E, Ye P, Shen W, Qian CG, Lin BF, Bickle QD (1998). Production and testing of *Schistosoma japonicum* candidate vaccine antigens in the natural ovine host. *Vaccine* 16: 1290-1298.

[71] McManus DP, Wong JY, Zhou J, Cai C, Zeng Q, Smyth D, Li Y, Kalinna BH, Duke MJ, Yi X (2001). Recombinant paramyosin (rec-Sj-97) tested for immunogenicity and vaccine efficacy against *Schistosoma japonicum* in mice and water buffaloes. *Vaccine* 20: 870-878.

[72] Chen HG, Nara T, Zeng XJ, Satoh M, Wu GC, Jiang WS, Yi FY, Kojima S, Zhang SJ, Hirayama K (2000). Vaccination of domestic pig with recombinant paramyosin against *Schistosoma japonicum* in China. *Vaccine* 18: 2142-2146.

[73] Shi F, Zhang Y, Ye P, Lin J, Cai Y, Shen W, Bickle QD, Taylor MG (2001). Laboratory and field evaluation of *Schistosoma japonicum* DNA vaccines in sheep and water buffalo in China. Vaccine 20: 462-467.

[74] Shi F, Zhang Y, Lin J, Zuo X, Shen W, Cai Y, Ye P, Bickle QD, Taylor MG (2002). Field testing of *Schistosoma japonicum* DNA vaccines in cattle in China. *Vaccine* 20: 3629-3631.

[75] Taylor MG, Huggins MC, Shi F, Lin J, Tian E, Ye P, Shen W, Qian CG, Lin BF, Bickle QD (1998). Production and testing of *Schistosoma japonicum* candidate vaccine antigens in the natural ovine host. *Vaccine* 16: 1290-1298.

[76] Xu S, Shi F, Shen W, Lin J, Wang Y, Ye P, Tian E, Qian C, Lin B, Shi Y (1995). Vaccination of sheep against *Schistosoma japonicum* with either glutathione S-transferase, keyhole limpet, haemocyanin or the freeze/thaw schistosomula/BCG vaccine. *Vet. Parasitol.* 58: 301-312.

[77] Liu SX, He YK, Song GC (1997). Anti-fecundity immunity to *Schistosoma japonicum* induced in Chinese water buffaloes (*Bos buffelus*) after vaccination with recombinant 26 kDa glutathione-S-transferase (reSjc26GST). *Vet. Parasitol.* 69: 39-47.

[78] Wu Z, Liu S, Zhang S, Tong H, Gao Z, Liu Y, Lin D, Liu Z, Wu G, Yi H, Song G, Xu Y (2004). Persistence of the protective immunity to *Schistosoma japonicum* in Chinese yellow cattle induced by recombinant 26 kDa glutathione-S-transferase (reSjc26GST). *Vet. Parasitol.* 123: 167-177.

[79] Liu SX, Song GC, Xu YX, Yang W, McManus DP (1995). Anti-fecundity immunity induced in pigs vaccinated with recombinant

Schistosoma japonicum 26 kDA glutathione-S-transferase. *Parasite Immunol.* 17: 335–340.

[80] Shi F, Lin J, Cai Y, Shen W. Taylor MG (1998). Evaluation on protective effects of three kinds of *Schistosoma japonicum* antigens against schistosomiasis in farm animals. In: Tada I, Kojima A, Tsuji M, ed. *Proceedings of the Ninth International Congress of Parasitology.* Bologna: Monduzzi Editore, 1217-1223.

[81] Liu JM, Cai XZ, Lin JJ, Fu ZQ, Yang GZ, Shi FH, Cai YM, Shen W, Taylor MG, Wu XF (2004). Gene cloning, expression and vaccine testing of *Schistosoma japonicum* SjFABPc. *Parasite Immunol* 26: 603-607.

[82] Zhu Y, Si J, Harn DA, Xu M, Ren J, Yu C, Liang Y, Yin X, He W, Cao G (2006). *Schistosoma japonicum* triose-phosphate isomerase plasmid DNA vaccine protects pigs against challenge infection. *Parasitology* 132: 67-71.

[83] Da'dara A, Li YS, Xiong T, Zhou J, Williams GM, McManus DP, Feng Z, Yu XL, Gray DJ, Harn DA (2008). DNA-based vaccines protect against zoonotic schistosomiasis in water buffalo. *Vaccine* 26(29-30): 3617-3625.

[84] Yu XL, He YK, Xiong T, Zhao YQ, Shi MZ, Zhou J, Liu ZC, Luo XS, Fu X, He HB, Harn DA, Li YS (2006). Protective effects of co-immunization with SjCTPI-Hsp70 and interleukin-12 DNA vaccines against *Schistosoma japonicum* challenge infection in water buffalo. *Zhongguo Ji Sheng Chong Xue Yu Ji Sheng Chong Bing Za Zhi.* 24(6): 433-436.

[85] Zhu Y, Ren J, Da'dara A, Harn D, Xu M, Si J, Yu C, Liang Y, Ye P, Yin X, He W, Xu Y, Cao G, Hua W (2004).The protective effect of a *Schistosoma japonicum* Chinese strain 23 kDa plasmid DNA vaccine in pigs is enhanced with IL-12. *Vaccine* 23(1): 78-83.

[86] McManus DP, Loukas A (2008). Current status of vaccines for schistosomiasis. *Clin. Microbiol. Rev.* 21(1): 225-242.

[87] Tang L, Zhou Z, Chen Y, Luo Y, Wang L, Chen L, Huang F, Zeng X, Yi X (2007). Vaccination of goats with 31 kDa and 32 kDa *Schistosoma japonicum* antigens by DNA priming and protein boosting. *Cell Mol. Immunol.* 4(2): 153-156.

[88] Scott JC, McManus DP (1999). Identification of novel 70-kDa heat shock protein from the human blood fluke of humans, *Schistosoma japonicum*. *Biochim. Biophys. Acta* 1517: 53-62.

[89] Xie LP, Shi YG, Han JJ, Ning CX, Deng WW (1998). Preliminary study on protective immunity against *Schistosoma japonicum* induced by different doses of naked DNA vaccine pCDSj32 in BALB/c mice. *Zhongguo Ji Sheng Chong Bing Fang Zhi Za Zhi* 11: 305-307.
[90] Yi XY, Zheng XF, Zheng XZ, Wan SP, Shu XH, Larry M (2000). Studies on anti-fecundity induced by cathepsin B DNA vaccine of *Schistosoma japonicum. Zhongguo Ren Shou Gong Fang Bing Za Zhi* 16: 45-47.
[91] Wang LD, Chen HG, Guo JG, Zeng XJ, Hong XL, Xiong JJ, Wu XH, Wang XH, Wang LY, Xia G, Hao Y, Chin DP, Zhou XN (2009). A strategy to control transmission of *Schistosoma japonicum* in China. *New Engl. J. Med.* 360: 121-128.
[92] Slingenbergh J, Gilbert M, de Balogh K, Wint W (2004). Ecological sources of zoonotic diseases. *Rev. Sci. Tech. Off Int. Epiz* 23: 467-484.
[93] One health initiative. http://onehealthinitiative.com

In: Schistosomiasis
Editor: Adriana Erica Miele ISBN: 978-1-63117-186-4

Chapter 6

Schistosomiasis in Pre-School Children in Sub-Saharan Africa: Epidemiology, Signs and Symptoms, Diagnosis, Treatment Options and the Challenges

Humphrey D. Mazigo[1,*], Rebecca Waihenya[2] and Domenica Morona[1]
[1]Department of Medical Parasitology and Entomology, School of Medicine, Catholic University of Health and Allied Sciences, Mwanza, Tanzania
[2]Department of Zoology, School of Biological Sciences, Jomo Kenyatta University of Agriculture and Technology, Nairobi, Kenya

Abstract

Classified among the neglected tropical diseases, schistosomiasis remains probably the most important of those occurring in sub-Saharan Africa.

* Corresponding author: Humphrey D. Mazigo. Department of Medical Parasitology and Entomology, School of Medicine, Catholic University of Health and Allied Sciences, P.O. Box 1464, Mwanza, Tanzania. E-mail: humphreymazigo@gmail.com.

The disease affects all age groups; mass drug administration (MDA) using praziquantel targeting population at risk is the major intervention measure against it. However, despite the fact that schistosomiasis affects pre-school children as young as 4-9 months-old and in some areas up to 78% of the pre-school children are infected by schistosomes, this age group is normally excluded from the MDA programmes. In addition, to date no published recommendation on the treatment of schistosomiasis in preschool-age children is available. This is mainly due to the lack of clinical trials data on the safety and efficacy of schistosomicides in this age group and to the fact that the extent of schistosomiasis in this group has not been fully appreciated. Thus pre-school children infected with schistosomes remain with the disease for 4-5 years before they can receive the first dose of praziquantel at primary school. The majority of these children suffer from severe morbidities related either to *S. mansoni* or *S. haematobium*. This chapter will cover the knowledge gap on the epidemiology of schistosomiasis, related morbidity (clinical signs and symptoms) and treatment options and its challenges, by reviewing the available evidence on epidemiology and treatment options of the disease in this age group.

Keywords: Schistosomiasis, pre-school children, growth impairment, treatment options, prevention

Introduction

A Brief Background

Schistosomiasis is a water-borne chronic parasitic disease known to be endemic in Africa since ancient times [3-7]. The schistosome parasite in humans was first described in 1851 in Egypt by the German physician Theodor Bilharz postmortem in the mesenteric veins of a patient [5, 6]. In 1902, another species was demonstrated by Sir Patrick Manson [8, 9], with eggs characterized by lateral spines in the stool of a West Indian patient [8, 9]. Sambon, in 1907, acknowledged the existence of two different species based on the morphology and origin of the eggs [10]. The life cycle of schistosomes was then demonstrated by Leiper in 1915 who confirmed the existence of the two distinct species, as argued by Manson in 1902 and Sambon in 1907-1909 [6-8]. The two species were further described to develop in different snail intermediate hosts, which belong not only to two different genera but also to different sub-families [6-8, 11].

The genus *Schistosoma* encompasses 19 species [13], but only five are of major public health concern to human. *Schistosoma haematobium* [13], causes urinary schistosomiasis, an important public health problem in 53 countries in Africa and in the Middle East [14-16]. *S. mansoni* [9, 10] causes intestinal and hepatic schistosomiasis, and is endemic in 54 countries worldwide, mostly in Africa [16, 17]. *Schistosoma japonicum* (discovered by Prof. Katsurada in 1904) causes intestinal and hepatic schistosomiasis, and is endemic in China, Indonesia, Thailand and The Philippines [16-19]. Two schistosome species have a focal distribution, *S. intercalatum* Fisher 1934, endemic in ten African countries, and *S. mekongi* occurring in Cambodia and Laos [17, 19].

The Biology of Schistosomes

The taxonomy of the genus Bilharzia was first described by Meckel Von Hemsbach in 1856 [12] and, in 1858 Weinland named the genus *Schistosoma,* of the family Schistosomatidae [13]. The members of the genus *Schistoma* are dioecious [13]. Adult schistosomes are white or grayish in colour with a cylindrical body. The body length varies between species (6–28 mm); males measure between 6–20 mm and females 10-30 mm. Both sexes possess oral and ventral suckers, the former opens into a blind digestive system. The suckers are used by the worms for attachment to the walls of the blood vessels. The outer teguments of the adult worms are complex and differ between sexes and species [1, 2]. The male schistosome is flat-leaf like and the body is folded to form a groove or gynaecophoric canal, in which the female worm resides. In the definitive host, the adult worms live in pairs and are found within the perivesical (for species causing uro-genital schistosomiasis) or mesenteric (for species causing intestinal and hepatic schistosomiasis) venous plexuses.

In general, schistosomes have a complex life cycle that alternates between the human definitive host and a freshwater molluscan intermediate host. In the definitive host, adult schistosomes are found in pairs within capillary blood vessels. After copulation (Figure 1), the females lay eggs in the peripheral branches of the capillary venules. Immature eggs pass through the vessels' wall aided by their spine and cytolytic secretions [20] and further develop in the lumen of the genitourinary tract, in the case of *S. haematobium,* or the intestine, in the case of *S. intercalatum* and *S. mansoni* [20]. Viable eggs are excreted with urine or faeces depending on the species and reach fresh water bodies, either by direct deposition in the water or by being washed in from a neighbouring deposition site.

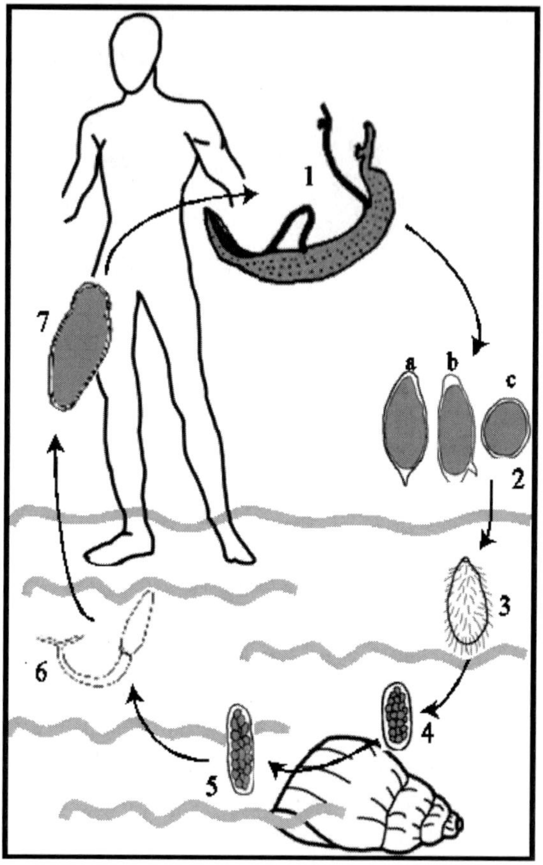

Figure 1. The life cycle of schistosomes, with a morphological description of the different life stages. Adult worms pair (1) living in the definitive human host blood (periportal veins for those species causing intestinal schistosomiasis; peri-bladder veins for those causing urogenital schistosomiasis). Each female lays 20-1000 eggs/day, depending on the species. The eggs (2) are recognizable by their morphology: (a) *S. haematobium* eggs present a terminal spine, (b) *S. mansoni* eggs have a lateral spine; (c) *S. japonicum* eggs are round with a rudimentary spine. The eggs are excreted by either faeces (b,c) or urine (a). Once they reach a freshwater source, they hatch into a free-living ciliated stage called miracidium (3). This one swims towards the mollusc host and penetrates it. Inside the freshwater snails asexual reproduction takes place to increase the number of parasites. Two sequential life stages arise from the miracidium: the mother (4) and the daughter sporocyst (5). This last releases into the water thousands of caudated free living cercariae (6), which are the infective stage for the human host. Cercariae are able to penetrate intact human skin and to develop into a juvenile form: the schistosomulum (7), which migrates undisturbed from the derma to the lungs, where it sexually matures into the adult form (1). The adults migrate to the final destination, where it can live for up to 30 years.

Under favourable conditions, the eggs hatch and release a larval stage known as miracidium [21]. For the continuation of the cycle, the miracidia will have to find the specific intermediate host within 8-12 hours (different species of snails act as intermediate hosts) [21]. They then penetrate the soft tissue of the snail and undergo some biological changes, transforming into mother sporocysts, which, in turn, asexually produce daughter sporocysts (Figure 1).

The daughter sporocysts migrate to the digestive glands of the snail and develop there into the bifurcated larval forms known as cercariae, which are infective to the definitive host [21-23]. After a variable incubation period (4-6 weeks) within the snails, free swimming, fork-tailed cercariae are released. On coming into contact with a susceptible host, the cercariae penetrate intact skin and transform into schistosomula [21-23], which enter the blood circulatory system, migrate to the liver and eventually to the bladder or mesenteries, where pairing of male and female schistosomes takes place, followed by a migration to the preferred sites of eggs deposition [22, 23]. *Schistosoma. haematobium* inhabits the terminal venules in the wall of the urinary bladder and the pelvic plexus and it causes urinary schistosomiasis, whereas *S. mansoni* inhabits the pericolon venules within the distribution of the portal venous system.

Epidemiology of Human Schistosomiasis in Sub-Saharan Africa

Classified among the neglected tropical diseases, schistosomiasis remains highly endemic and is the cause of chronic morbidities in Sub-Saharan Africa [24, 25].

In this region, both urogenital and intestinal schistosomiasis, caused by infection with *S. haematobium*, *S. intercalatum* and *S. mansoni* are highly endemic [24-26]. *S. haematobium* and *S. mansoni* are the most widely distributed and cause the greatest burden of morbidity and mortality [24-26]. Of the estimated 207 million individuals infected with schistosomiasis, 93% (192 million individuals) occurs in Sub-Saharan Africa [24, 25, 27]. It is estimated that two-thirds of the cases which occur in the region are caused by *S. haematobium*, an important causal agent of urinary tract disease [24, 29]. Due to its focal distribution, *S. mansoni,* the causative agent of intestinal disease, is responsible only for one-third of the human schistosomiasis cases in the same region [24]. The estimated disability-adjusted life years (DALYs) due to schistosomiasis range between 1.7-4.5 millions DALYs lost annually;

in Sub-Saharan Africa alone, the estimation ranges between 1.6-4.2 million DALYs [24].

However, these figures have been criticized for underestimating the true picture of the disease burden of schistosomiasis [30].

The transmission of the disease is influenced by a number of factors, all playing an important role: (i) the distribution, biology and population dynamics of the intermediate snail hosts [31, 32]; (ii) the patterns and extent of environmental contamination with human excreta, which in turn determine the prevalence and intensity of infection in human [31, 33]; (iii) the socio-economic and hygienic backgrounds of the affected population [34]; (iv) the host-parasite relationships, in both the snail and human hosts; and (v) protective mechanisms in the human host [35]. Thus, in endemic areas of tropical and sub-tropical regions, people get infected because they lack access to safe, potable water and maintain the transmission due to poor disposal systems and a continued contact with infested water through farming, domestic and recreational activities (Figure 2).

In the affected areas, Schistosomiasis affects individuals of all age groups. The highest prevalence, intensity and morbidity occurs in school-aged children, adolescents and young adults [36].

Traditionally, the prevalence and infection intensity gets to peak among children aged 10 to 15 years old [28, 37]. Conversely, a high occupational exposure associated with fishing or farming may result into the maintenance of high intensities of infection in adult individuals [38]. Children are particularly important as reservoirs of the infection due to their indiscriminate excretory habits, especially urination, when swimming and their unrivalled opportunities for water contacts in hot climates (Figure 3) [19, 32, 39].

Epidemiology of Schistosomiasis in Pre-School Aged Children

Prevalence and Intensity of Human Schistosomiasis

It is worthwhile to note that, though the occurrence of human schistosomiasis in pre-school aged children was noted since the 1950's [40], the focus on the epidemiology and morbidities associated with the disease in that particular age group is only a recent research development [40-44].

Most of the control programmes designed to date mainly focus on school-aged children (>7 years), overlooking younger children, regardless of the fact that pre-school children are also exposed to transmission sites (Figure 3) [45, 46], get infected and remain at risk of developing morbidity in early childhood [47]. An additional reason not to consider that age group may have been rooted in the assumption that those children have very little direct contact with water infested by schistosomes' cercariae. Furthermore, the lack of data on the safety of anti-schistosomal drugs in younger age groups at that time, as well as the high cost of the drugs may have prevented a wider coverage of the population in the control programs, with the inclusion of preschool children [47-49].

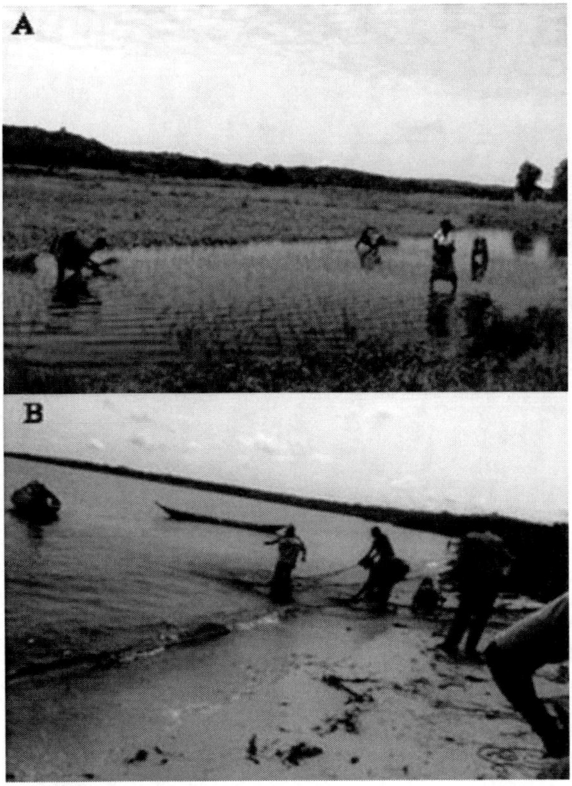

Courtesy of Mazigo HD.

Figure 2. Economic activities such as paddy cultivation and fishing increase the risk of transmission of schistosomiasis in Sub-Saharan Africa. Panel A: Paddy cultivation in flooded areas and Panel B: fishing along the southern shore of Lake Victoria basin, North-Western Tanzania.

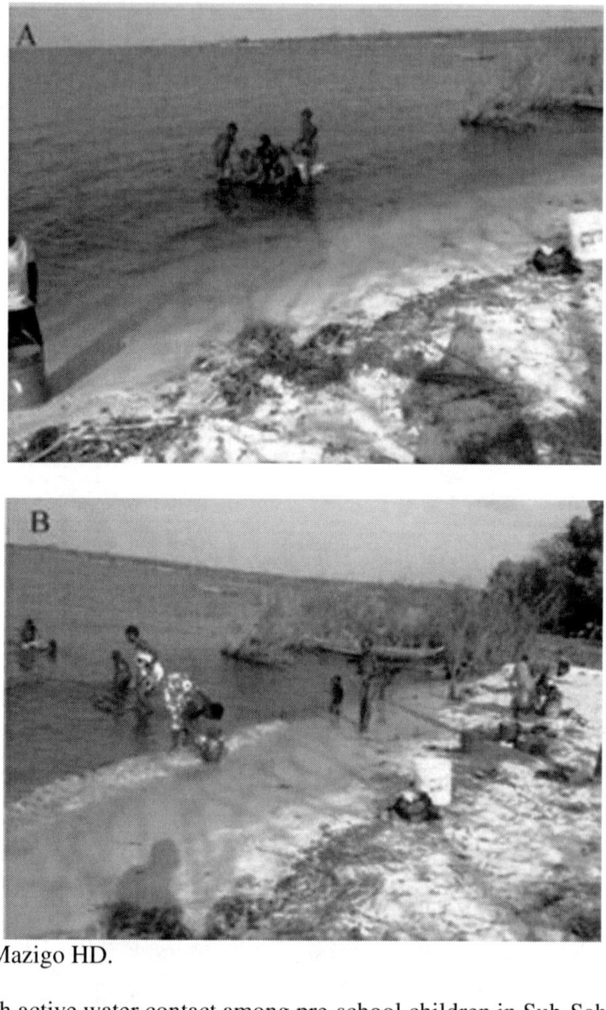

Courtesy of Mazigo HD.

Figure 3. High active water contact among pre-school children in Sub-Saharan Africa increases the risk of transmission of schistosomiasis in pre-school-aged children. Pre-school children bathing (Panel A) and swimming (Panel B) along the shore of the southern shore of the Lake Victoria, North-Western Tanzania.

It has been recently acknowledged that transmission of schistosomiasis in pre-school children is a serious public health concern in Sub-Saharan Africa [47-49]. Evidence from Uganda, Kenya, Zimbabwe, Ghana, Mali, Niger, Nigeria, Zanzibar and Sudan clearly indicates that schistosomes' infections occur in children as young as 4-9 months of age [47-64].

As described by Stothard et al. [64] an absolute age of first infections and the accumulated risk of infection are difficult to define as exposure patterns vary enormously, the authors rather define a "window of exposure" [64].

The pre-school age group is undoubtedly living at risk of both urogenital and intestinal schistosomiasis and some of the children harbour a high infection intensity, i.e., up to 7,284 eggs per gram of faeces for *S. mansoni* [65]. The high intensity of infection observed in pre-school children may already imply important health consequences. Without an early treatment and with a continual exposure to risk areas and a repeated exposure to the parasites, the risk of developing a significant morbidity as children grow up will be increased. Table 1 summarizes the available evidence on the prevalence and intensity of human schistosomiasis in pre-school children in Sub-Saharan Africa.

The prevalence of schistosomiasis in pre-school children varies from one geographical area to another. The wide distribution of *S. haematobium* in the region accounts for a high prevalence of the disease in this age group. For instance, Niger, Mali and Nigeria are known to be highly endemic regions for *S. haematobium* [49-64] and studies in this age group (<7 years), have reported high prevalences, ranging from 15% to 71.8% [51, 55, 56, 58]. For *S. mansoni*, the prevalence varied from 7% to 85.7% [59-64]. The geographical variation in prevalence is partly, associated with variations in the exposure to risk factors, the type and sensitivity of the tests used and the endemicity of the disease [50-64].

The prevalence observed increases with the increase in age of the children, within the age group 4-5 years old recording the highest values [50-64]. Probably, children at this age are more extensively and permanently exposed to cercariae in the water than those of 1-2 years old [56]. The observed pattern of increase in prevalence with age is common in Sub-Saharan Africa [36]. In school-going children, the prevalence has been observed to peak between 10-19 years and to decrease thereafter with increasing age [36]. Therefore a thorough representation of the age-dependent pattern of infection for *S. haematobium* would peak around 5-19 year-old age group and decreases in the age group > 20 years old [36].

In Sub-Saharan Africa, due to the wide distribution and high endemicity of the two forms of the disease, co-infection of urogenital and intestinal schistosomiasis does occur in all age groups and equally in pre-school children [55, 66]. In the latter group, co-infection of *S. mansoni* and *S. haematobium* has been reported in endemic areas of Sierra Leone and Cote d'Ivoire, with a recorded prevalence of 29% [55, 66].

This has clinical and public health implications, as pre-school children will most of the time remain untreated for both infections until they start their primary school education. In addition, the interaction between *S. haematobium* and *S. mansoni* infections and other tropical diseases such as malaria, soil transmitted helminths and bacterial infections, such as *Mycobacterium tuberculosis,* has not been thoroughly investigated and requires more research.

The majority of the pre-school (≤ 6 years) children in endemic areas for intestinal schistosomiasis have a light intensity of infection (<100 epg) and only few show a high intensity (≥ 400 epg) [59-64]. The age group 4-5 years old shows a higher intensity of infection [59-64]. There is a significant association between a heavy infection intensity and the risk of developing schistosomiasis-related morbidities. For instance, a heavy intensity of infection with *S. mansoni* is associated with a risk of bloody diarrhoea, anaemia, undernutrition, hepatosplenomegaly and structural urinary tract diseases [60]. A direct relationship between the intensity of infection and the abnormalities of the urinary tract has been observed, whereby calcified urinary bladder, deformed ureters and hydronephrosis have been reported in school-aged children with high infection intensities (excreted >250 eggs/10 ml of urine) [67-70]. In addition, the development of an immunoregulatory inflammatory response against the trapped eggs determines the risk of organomegaly morbidities [71]. However, in endemic areas, a light intensity of infection should not be overlooked as a cause of schistosome-related morbidities [72].

Risk Factors Associated with the Exposure of Pre-School Children to Human-Schistosomiasis

Various factors have been described which may increase the risk of infection for pre-school children at a very early stage in their life [51, 55, 58, 63]. In endemic areas, pre-school children are exposed to cercariae-infested water sources when they accompany their guardians/caregivers/mothers to the transmissions sites (Figure 4) [63]. In many areas of Sub-Saharan Africa, Focus Group Discussions (FGDs) have been conducted to generate information on water contact behaviour among pre-school children and have revealed that water contact, particularly for children <2 years old, was due to their mothers activities along the shores of water sources, such as washing, bathing and fishing [51, 55, 58]. Passive transmission of schistosomiasis to infants also occurs through bathing of the children with cercariae-infested water along the shores of water sources (Figure 4).

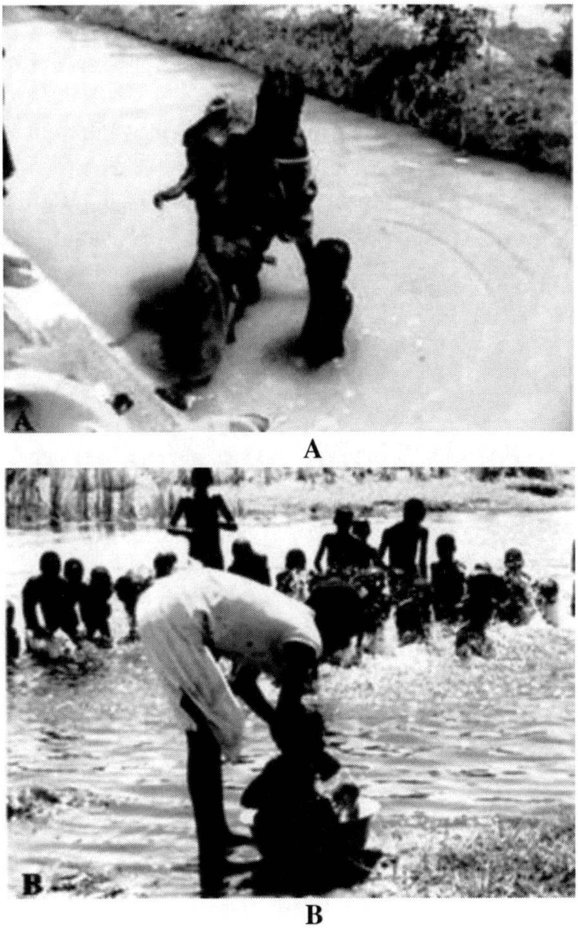

Reproduced with permission from [55].

Figure 4. Active and passive water contact increases the risks for schistosomiasis transmission in pre-school children: mothers bathing their children in a canal (Panel A) and in a small bucket while other children are playing in the water sources in Niger (Panel B).

The older children (>5 yrs) have been observed or have admitted visiting water sources for bathing, washing, fetching water, swimming and fishing (Figures 3 and 4) [51, 58]. In Niger, observation studies have reported that up to 69.8% of the pre-school children accompanied their mothers to schistosomiasis active transmission sites before their first birthday and that the majority of the mothers used water directly drawn from the schistosomiasis-infested water sources to bath their children [55].

In other endemic areas, children taken to the lake shore by their mothers remained five times more at risk of being infected, while children whose mothers were infected with *S. mansoni* were almost six times more likely to be infected. The older children who spent more time in water sources remained at higher risk of being infected [73].

Moreover, the lack of an appropriate waste disposal system in some of the endemic communities is an additional factor for a high and continuous transmission of the disease in all age groupsIt is also worth mentioning that an early exposure of the pre-school children to the disease may lead to the early development of schistosomiasis morbidity, if left untreated [71, 74].

Clinical Signs and Morbidity

i. Signs and Symptoms of Human Schistosomiasis in Pre-School Children

The clinical signs and symptoms observed or reported in pre-school children may not differ from the ones observed in other age groups living in endemic areas.

However, the extent and severity of the disease in this age group could lead to a high morbidity due to the slow development of acquired immunity against the parasites. Following infection, acute and chronic clinical signs and symptoms of the disease may gradually occur.

ii. Early Manifestation

Early signs characterized by skin reactions following penetration of the cercariae larval stage may occur in infected individuals; however, these manifestations rarely occur among the residents of schistosomiasis endemic areas [75, 76].

In sensitized non-resident individuals of endemic areas, rashes may appear following the penetration of the cercariae and can persist for up to one week [75-77].

iii. Katayama Fever (Acute Schistosomiasis)

Though this is quite a rare sign of the disease for residents of endemic areas [78-80], the symptom is common in areas of high transmission and results from the immune response against the eggs of the parasites deposited in the hosts' tissues. Katayama fever is mainly characterized by fever, headache, myalgia, right-upper quadrant pain, bloody diarrhoea and respiratory symptoms [78-80].

Other reported clinical signs and symptoms include hepatomegaly and splenomegaly, and a full blood picture examination reveals eosinophilia [78-80].

iv. Chronic Schistosomiasis

For both intestinal and urogenital schistosomiasis, the chronic stage of the disease results from the host's immune response against the hepatotoxins-Omega-1 released from the trapped eggs in the tissues [81, 82]. The immune response is characterized by a type IV hypersensitivity reaction mediated through T-helper cells (Th_2) directed against the egg antigens [83, 84]. The chronic immune reaction eventually leads to the formation of granulomas which destroy the trapped eggs; however, it may also lead to the deposition of fibrotic tissues in the hosts tissues [83, 84]. The majority of the formed granuloma tissues develop at the sites of maximal accumulation of eggs [83, 84]. The development of granulomas depends on host and parasite genetics [85], the degree and length of exposure [86], the intensity of infection [87], the host immune response to the parasite and the co-infection with other tropical diseases, such as malaria and HIV [88].

Chronic Intestinal Schistosomiasis

The predilection sites of adult *S. mansoni* being the mesenteric veins, the laid eggs transverse the intestinal wall of the large bowel inducing inflammation, ulceration, polyposis and micro-abscess formation [89, 90]. In mild infections, pre-school children may present with diarrhoea, abdominal pain, bloody stool, constipation, nausea and drowsiness [60, 91]. In pre-school children, diarrhoea, blood in stool or occult blood, are common and correlate strongly with intestinal schistosomiasis [60]. Generally, severe chronic intestinal schistosomiasis may result into colonic or rectal stenosis, which may manifest as protein-loosing enteropathy [71].

The trapped eggs in the mucosa or other parts of the body are swept by the portal blood flow and accumulate in the presinusoidal venules within the portal triads [89, 90]. The immunological response against the eggs antigens may result into the development of extensive fibrosis in the liver, leading to hepatomegaly or splenomegaly or hepatosplenomegaly, venous obstructions, portal hypertension and the development of oesophageal varices [89, 90]. In pre-school children, hepatomegaly, splenomegaly and hepatosplenomegaly may occur following an early infection with schistosomes, which remained untreated for 4-5 years [74].

In addition, obstructions of the large or small intestine have been reported in pre-school children infected with *S. mansoni* [92].

Chronic Urogenital Schistosomiasis

The adult worms of *S. haematobium* are located within the terminal venules surrounding the urinary bladder, thus enhancing the passage of the laid eggs into the lumen of the urinary bladder, pelvic organs and other gastrointestinal organs [93]. Eggs trapped in the wall of the urinary bladder provoke immunological responses, which lead to the formation of granulomas primarily affecting the ureter [93].

The immunological response may also lead to the formation of sandy patches, ulcerations and polypoid lesions along the urinary bladder wall and ureters, resulting into haematuria, obstruction of the urine flow, calcified bladder wall and cancer [96]In pre-school children, micro and macro-haematuria accompanied with dysuria are the early and late signs of an established disease (those signs appear within 10-12 weeks of infection) [51, 53, 54, 58].

The late manifestations associated with urogenital schistosomiasis include proteinuria, calcification in the bladder, obstruction of the ureter, renal colic, hydronephrosis and renal failure [93, 94].

On ultrasonographical examination, children have been observed to have structural abnormalities of the urinary bladder and ureters [93, 94].

The development of urological abnormalities related to *S. haematobium* infection is associated with the intensity of infection [67, 68, 71].

v. Anaemia, Stunted Growth and Cognitive Function

Both intestinal and urogenital schistosomiasis have been associated with anaemia, stunted growth and poor cognitive functions in children [71, 95-97].

Studies have confirmed the relationship between anaemia and schistosomiasis, even after adjustment for co-infections and dietary factors [71, 98].

Intestinal schistosomiasis causes anaemia through blood loss in stool (feacal occult blood) resulting from the penetration of the eggs through the intestinal wall into the gastrointestinal lumen [71, 96, 98, 99], while *S. haematobium* causes anaemia through haematuria and proteinuria [100]. In Uganda, a prevalence of 68.9% of anaemia, with 3.7% of the children having severe anaemia, was recorded in pre-school children [98].

Many of these children were co-infected with intestinal schistosomiasis and *Plasmodium falciparum* malaria [98]. Anaemia appears to be common in pre-school children carrying a high intensity of infection [98].

Increasing evidence suggests that schistosomiasis infection in childhood is associated with stunted growth, malnutrition, and poor cognitive functions, even at a light intensity of infection [71, 101]. In Tanzania, school-aged children infected with schistosomiasis also presented with stunted growth [102]. Increased hepatic fibrosis has been significantly associated with under-nutrition, and a heavy intensity of infection, with the risk of stunted growth [71].

Moreover, a heavy infection with *S. haematobium* has been associated with impaired mental performances or poor cognitive function [103]. Evidence from clinical studies indicates that a successful chemotherapy leads to a substantial improvement of the haemoglobin level but to an incomplete catch-up in growth [104, 105].

To date, most of the studies on the effects of schistosomiasis on haemoglobin levels, growth and cognitive functions have focused on school-aged children, however, recently, the possible effects of schistosomes on stunting, cognitive functions and haemoglobin levels in pre-school children have been researched upon [98]. Early infection in pre-school children as young as 4-9 months may give rise to the development of advanced morbidities related to schistosomiasis at the early age of 4-5 years and may become more serious at older ages.

These morbidities cannot be entirely reversed following chemotherapy. For example, an early infection with schistosomiasis could have an impact on the cognitive development and functions of the infected pre-school children, which is not reversible with chemotherapy. In school-aged children, improvement of growth was not significant at 18 months following treatment [101].

Diagnosis of Schistosomiasis in Pre-School Children

Direct Eggs Detection Methods

Quantitative and qualitative diagnostic techniques are recommended for the diagnosis of schistosomiasis, either in older age groups or in pre-school children [106-109].

The observation of the eggs characteristics (with lateral spines for *S. mansoni* or terminal spines for *S. haematobium*, Figure 1) in stool or urine samples confirms the diagnosis [106].

The World Health Organization recommends the use of the standardized thick smear (41.7 mg) Kato Katz technique, which is regarded as a gold standard for the diagnosis of *S. mansoni* in routine epidemiological surveys and population-based surveys [106].

According to the WHO guidelines, the intensity of infection is classified as: 'negative' (no eggs observed); 'light infection intensity' (1-99 eggs per gram of faeces (epg), 'medium infection' (100-399 epg) and 'heavy intensity of infection' (≥ 400 epg) [106]. For *S. haematobium* infection, urine filtration methods and direct parasitological examination are used to determine the infection status and intensity, in which the infection level is classified as 'infection negative' (no eggs observed), 'light intensity of infection' (1-49 eggs/ 10 ml of urine) and 'heavy intensity of infection' (≥ 50 eggs/10 ml of urine) [106]. Due to the circadian pattern of eggs' excretion, urine specimens should ideally be collected between 10 am and 2 pm, and preferably after physical exercise [106].

Other diagnostic techniques that can be used in research or in clinical practices are concentrations methods (formol-ether concentration technique, FLOTAC, Percoll and direct wet preparation) [64].

The intensity of infection in pre-school children is usually low (light intensity of infection), hence using Kato Katz and urine filtration methods may miss out the infection due to the low sensitivity of these techniques, particularly in detecting light intensity of infections [64, 106].

In addition, the immunity of the host influences the ability to excrete eggs in infected individual and may affect the sensitivity of these tests, as individuals with low immunity may retain more eggs and excrete only few in stool or urine [64].

Probably, in infected pre-school children, the immunity against the parasite may still be developing and the eggs' excretion efficiency may be poor, leading to false negative results when only urine and stool samples are used for diagnosis [64, 110]. Thus, combining quantitative and qualitative methods for the diagnosis of schistosomiasis in pre-school children is important.

Antigen Based Diagnostic Techniques

To overcome the challenges of the Kato Katz and other direct detection techniques, qualitative diagnostic methods have been developed and are being used for clinical and epidemiological population-based surveys on *S. mansoni* and *S. haematobium* [64, 107-109, 111]. Depending on the migratory characteristics in the electrophoresis, two kits are available, the Circulating Anodic Antigens (CAA) and the Circulating Cathodic Antigen (CCA) immune-chromatographic kits, which detect the presence of feeding adult worms by detecting excreted schistosomes antigens in the host urine [64, 107-109, 111]. The sensitivity and specificity of the tests have been evaluated in pre-school children [64, 107-109, 111] and the tests provided similar results to quantitative techniques but with an increased detection rate of positive cases [64, 107-109, 111]. Recently, a new rapid diagnostic test, which combines both *S. mansoni* and *S. haematobium,* has been introduced in the field [108, 111]. For a single evaluation in the field, the sensitivity of the test was 75% against Kato Katz techniques and, when compared with urine filtration techniques, the sensitivity was 66.7% [111]. However, the specificity of the rapid test when the eggs detection techniques were used as reference standard was 34.4% [111].

Antibodies Based Tests

Antibodies-based techniques have also been developed for diagnosis; commercially available ELISA kits which use finger-prick blood samples to detect schistosome adult worm protein (SAWP) have been explored in endemic areas, particularly in pre-school children [52, 61, 64]. However, these techniques cannot distinguish active from past infections with a long-term persistence of the parasites antigen after chemotherapy and the inability to measure the infection intensity.

Molecular Diagnosis

The Polymerase Chain Reaction (PCR) technique for detection of *S. mansoni* has been explored [113, 114] and the technique has proven to be highly sensitive in areas of light and medium intensity infection. However, the technique has limited use in endemic areas due to its high cost [115]. Detailed information on various diagnostic techniques of intestinal schistosomiasis in pre-school children are discussed by Stothard and colleagues in East Africa [64].

Diagnosis of Schistosomiasis-Related Morbidities

For *S. haematobium*, the presence of macro-haematuria is an indicator of an active infection and acts as a sign of urinary bladder damage. Indirect diagnostic tests are used such as Urine Reagent Strips (Multistix) which detect blood in urine (micro-macro haematuria); the characterization of other urine chemical/physical properties are also used for epidemiological surveys [116, 117]. Urine-albumin levels in urine are measured using the Albumin-HemoCue photometer [117]. Macro-haematuria and urine turbidity are assessed visually and quantified with the use of a bar-coded chart [117].

A questionnaire-based method to ascertain the occurrence/history of haematuria was developed by the Red Urine Study supported by the WHO [118, 119].

The usefulness and sensitivity of the questionnaire for estimating the prevalence among school children has been demonstrated [118, 119].

Organ-specific morbidities related to *S. mansoni* (hepatomegaly, splenomegaly, hepatosplenomegaly and portal fibrosis) and to *S. haematobium* (urinary tract pathologies, calcified urinary bladder, calcified and distorted ureters, hydronephrosis and non-functioning kidney) [90, 91, 94] are diagnosed using ultrasonography in population-based surveys or in clinical practices [90, 91, 94].

Unfortunately, the ultrasonography technique requires expensive equipments, is time-consuming, has a low sensitivity to mild lesions early inflammatory changes, and presents inter-and-intra observers variations in scoring the observed pathology [117].

Treatment of Schistosomiasis and Its Challenges in Pre-School Children

The WHO recommends regular de-worming of children and other specialgroups at risk of infection [120]The approach used is Mass Drug Administration (MDA) using praziquantel (40 mg/kg) for controlling schistosomiasis-related morbidities, especially among school aged-children (6-15 years) and among high-risk adults (>15 years old), i.e., fishermen/women [120]. For school-aged children, the approach mainly uses school resources and targets the children with heavy infection [120]. The approach is regarded as cost-effective [120], as the drug used is safe, highly efficacious, cheap and can reverse most of the schistosomiasis-related morbidities, in particular at the early stages of the disease [121-123]. However, this approach has been criticized for overlooking schistosomes' infections in other groups of the community, especially the pre-school children, who, as assumed, have an insufficient risk of exposure and, therefore may have a light infection intensity, often regarded as insignificant in terms of the development of a clinical disease [71].

In addition, lack of or limited documentation on the safety of anti-schistosomes drugs in the younger age group is among the reasons to exclude this particular group from mass treatment [40, 45, 46, 50]. However, numerous studies have now confirmed that many of the pre-school aged children living in areas with high transmission of schistosomiasis in sub-Saharan Africa are actually infected and several trials on the efficacy and side effects of praziquantel in pre-school school children have been conducted [18-22]. Table 2 summarizes the results of clinical trials on the efficacy and side effects of praziquantel at a dose of 40 mg/kg in pre-school children in sub-Saharan Africa.

Praziquantel is the drug of choice for the treatment and morbidity control of schistosomiasis. Easy administration, good tolerability and low price are important features of this drug that contribute to its extensive use in the control of schistosomiasis in sub-Saharan Africa [50].

Treatment of schistosomiasis in pre-school and school-going children has the effect to reverse impaired growth, improve cognitive function, reverse the early organomegaly and other morbidities [50].

Moreover, the death of adults schistosomes following treatment stimulates the immune responses and boosts the antibody responses which are associated with protection against re-infection [124].

Previous data have indicated cure rates ranging from 75 to 85% for *S. haematobium*; from 63 to 85% for *S. mansoni* and, from 60 to 80% for mixed infection of *S. mansoni* and *S. haematobium* [23, 70, 94, 125, 126].

Results from clinical trials conducted among pre-school children between 2000 and 2013 indicate that the cure rates of praziquantel in this age group were high, with a significant reduction in mean egg counts (Egg Reduction Rates-ERR) for both *S. haematobium* and *S. mansoni,* signifying that the treatment is likely to avert the development of a chronic morbidity at older ages [41, 44, 48, 56, 65, 66, 73].

It should also be noted that, there are geographical variations in cure rates and eggs reduction rates reported in pre-school children. In Zimbabwe, among children infected with *S. haematobium,* high cure and eggs reduction rates were observed (cure rate 92% and egg reduction rate 99%) [41, 44, 48, 56, 65, 66, 73], while in Uganda, among children infected with *S. mansoni*, the overall cure rate was 56.4%, with lower cure rates observed in children who had previously received praziquantel treatment (cure rate CR 41.9%) [65].

In Uganda, the factors associated with the cure rate (egg negative after praziquantel treatment) were age (e.g., children less than 3 years having a lower cure rate), light infections (e.g., heavily infected children having a lower cure rate) and no history of praziquantel treatment (e.g., children having a history of praziquantel treatment recording a lower cure rate) [65].

Several assumptions were made on the reasons for the low cure rates observed among pre-school children, including a lower anti-worm immune response in this age group, sensitivity to praziquantel, which is dependent on the maturity of the parasites and the fact that younger children may have a high proportion of immature worms, not eliminated by praziquantel [41, 65].

Only mild and transient side effects of the praziquantel treatment are reported in the younger age group. Most of them occur within the first four hours after treatment and gradually resolve within 24 hours. Some of the side effects are associated with the presence and intensity of the adult worms in the body [41, 44, 48, 56, 65, 66, 73].

It is worth to note that the host body immunity can only recognize the dying adult schistosmes as an antigen and this may provoke a strong immune response leading to allergic reactions in some of the treated pre-school children [124]. The majority of the reported side effects are alike (Table 2). In general, praziquantel (40 mg/kg or 60 mg/kg) remains a safe drug for the treatment of schistosomiasis (both *S. mansoni* and *S. haematobium*) in pre-school children.

Table 1. Prevalence and intensity of infection of schistosomiasis in pre-school children in Sub-Saharan Africa

Region	Country	Geographical area	Schistosome species	Major findings (prevalence and intensity of infection)	Reference
West Africa	Nigeria	Ogun State	*S. haematobium*	A total of 209 preschool children aged < 5 years were screened, 150/209 (71.8%: 72.4% in boys and 70.9% in girls) had infection. 62.7% of the children had light infection (<50 eggs/10 mls urine) and 9.6% (≥ 50 eggs/10 mls) had heavy infection. Only 17.7% of the children had visible haematuria.	[51]
	Ghana	Awutu-Efutu Senya District	*S. haematobium*	A total of 97 preschool children aged between 20 months and 5 years were included in the study. Prevalence of *S. haematobium* by MoAb-dipstick was 30% and by microscopy was 11.2%. The intensity of infection for 9 children who were microscopy positive ranged from 1-222 eggs/10 mls of urine with majority having light infection of 1-10 eggs/10 ml and 32 eggs/10 ml. Only one child had heavy infection (≥ 50 eggs/10 ml of urine): 222 eggs/ml.	[52]
	Nigeria	Adim	*S. haematobium*	A total of 126 preschool children aged 0-5 years were examined for urogenital schistosomiasis; the overall prevalence was 19.8% (25/126), boys had 21.1% and girls 18.2% with infection being common in the age group 2-5 years. Both prevalence and intensity of infection increased with age, with the highest infection rate of 26.8% in the 5 year-old children. The overall geometric mean egg count was 5.9 eggs/10 ml urine with no significant difference between boys (6.2 eggs/10 ml urine) and girls (5.6 eggs/10 ml urine). Absolute eggs counts ranged from 1-25 eggs/10 ml urine A total of 32.5% and 27.8% of the children had haematuria and proteinuria.	[53]

Table 1. (Continued)

Region	Country	Geographical area	Schistosome species	Major findings (prevalence and intensity of infection)	Reference
West Africa	Nigeria	Abeokuta	*S. haematobium*	A total of 213 preschool children were enrolled in a study and only 167 submitted urine samples (age 1-6 years). Overall prevalence of *S. haematobium* was 58.1% (boys 57.1% and girls 59.2%) with children aged 4 years having the highest prevalence (69.2%). The geometrical mean intensity of infection was 1.17 eggs/10 ml of urine with children aged 3 years having the highest mean intensity of infection of 1.34 eggs/10 mls of urine. The overall prevalence of microhaematuria was 47.4%.	[54]
	Niger	Falmado and Diambala	*S. haematobium* and *S. mansoni*	A total of 282 pre-school children aged <5 years were enrolled in the study. The overall prevalence of *S. haematobium* was 60.5% in Diambala and 50.5% in Falmado (with no sex differences). Prevalence of heavy infection (≥ 50 eggs/10 ml of urine) was 6.2% in Falmado. The prevalence of macro and microhaematuria was respectively 5.2% and 50.5% in Falmado and 2.2% and 38.9% in Diambala	[55]
				The overall prevalence of *S. mansoni* was 43.8% with no sex differences. Almost 17.3% of the children a had light infection (1-99 epg), 23.8% had a moderate infection (100-399 epg) and 2.7% had a heavy infection (≥ 400 epg).	
				In Diambala, 28.6% of the children were co-infected with *S. mansoni* and *S. haematobium*.	

Region	Country	Geographical area	Schistosome species	Major findings (prevalence and intensity of infection)	Reference
West Africa	Mali	Sahelian rural	*S. haematobium*	A total of 338 preschool children aged 1- 4 years were examined. The overall prevalence was 51.2% (173/338) with no sex differences. However, the age group 4 years had the highest prevalence, 53.6%. The overall prevalence of heavy infection was (≥ 50 eggs/ml) 15.7% where majority of the children had light infection (≤ 50 eggs/10 ml of urine) 35.5%. The geometric mean intensity of infection was 18.41 eggs/10 ml of urine (13.59-24.92 eggs/10 ml of urine). The highest mean intensity of infection was observed in 4 years age group at 25.78 eggs/10 ml of urine	[56]
	Sierra Leone	Bo, Kailahun, Kenema, Koinadugu, Kono, Tonkolili and other hard to reach rural villages	*S. mansoni*	The study included a total of 1803 preschool children aged 4-5 years. The overall prevalence of *S. mansoni* after 3 phases of screening was 11.2% and arithmetic mean intensity of infections was 33.5 epg with sex differences. The district located on the coastal areas had no cases of *S. mansoni.*	[57]
	Nigeria	Korede and Obada, Ijebu East Ogun State	*S. haematobium*	Of the 100 pre-school children aged ≤ 1 to ≤ 6 years only 83 of them submitted stool samples for screening. The overall prevalence was 16.9% (18.4% in boys and 14.7% in girls). The geometric mean intensity of infection was 0.149 eggs/10 ml of urine. The age group 5-6 years had highest mean intensity of infection (0.268 eggs/10 ml). The prevalence of microhaematuria was 48.2%.	[58]

Table 1. (Continued)

Region	Country	Geographical area	Schistosome species	Major findings (prevalence and intensity of infection)	Reference
East Africa	Uganda	Mayuge and Bugiri districts	*S. mansoni*	Survey I: a total of 136 pre-school children aged < 3 years were included. Overall prevalence of *S. mansoni* was 7% with one participant having 156 eggs/g of faeces. Majority of the children had light intensity (≤100 eggs/gram of faeces). Based on the Circulating Cathodic Antigens (CCA) results, the prevalence was 40%. Survey II: A total of 19 pre-school children (aged <3 years) were included in the study. The prevalence of egg-patent *S. mansoni* infections was 85.7% at Bugoto and 25% at Bwondha. All of the children had light intensity of infection (≤ 100 epg). Based on CCA, 50% of children from Bwondha were positive for *S. mansoni*. In general, the overall prevalence of *S. mansoni* was 47.4%.	[59]
	Uganda	Buliisa district (Bugoigo, Walukuba and Piida villages)	*S. mansoni*	A total of 572 pre-school children aged 4 months to 6.5 years were recruited into the study. The overall prevalence of *S. mansoni* was 27.2% (geometric mean 1.9 epg and arithmetic mean of intensity of infection was 47.62 epg).	[60]
	Kenya	Usoma, Kisumu	*S. mansoni*	A study involved pre-school children aged 1-5 years. A total of 216 children were recruited and the overall prevalence was 37%. For intensity of infection of *S. mansoni,* 24 (63%) had low-intensity of infection, 9 (24%) had moderate-intensity and 5 913%) had heavy-intensity of infection.	[61]

Region	Country	Geographical area	Schistosome species	Major findings (prevalence and intensity of infection)	Reference
East Africa	Uganda	Buliisa district	*S. mansoni*	1,028 pre-school aged ≤ 6 years were recruited into the study. The prevalence of *S. mansoni* in children from Lake Albert was 45.9% and those from Lake Victoria was 40.7%. The geometric mean for children from Lake Albert was 5.5epg and mean epg was 230.8. For children from Lake Victoria, the geometric mean was 6.7 and mean epg was 477.7. The proportion of children severely infected (≥ 400 epg) was higher for children from the Lake Victoria, 11.6% compared to 5.5%.	[62]
	Uganda	Bugoigo	*S. mansoni*	A total of 36 pre-school children aged <6 years were recruited. At baseline, the overall prevalence was 67% and majority of them had light intensity of infection (< 100 epg, 72%), moderate intensity of infection (100-399 epg, 20%) and heavy intensity of infection (≥ 400 epg, 8%).	[63]
	Uganda	Bugoigo	*S. mansoni*	A total of 242 pre-school children were included in the study. The prevalence of *S. mansoni* based on direct egg-detection methods in stools, schistosomes antigens in urine (CCA), Antibodies to soluble egg antigen were 24.4%, 42.6% and 45.9%. The overall prevalence based on Kato Katz was 21.9% and the mean epg (of positive) was 86.4 epg. 16.9% of the children had light intensity of infection (<100 epg), 4.5 % had moderate intensity (100-399 epg) and 0.4% had heavy intensity. The age at first detection of *S. mansoni* using different diagnostic techniques ranged from 9 months to 2 years.	[64]

Table 2. Results of clinical trials of praziquantel in pre-school children: efficacy of praziquantel treatment and side effects

Country	Species	Efficacy of Praziquantel (PZQ) treatment (cure rates and egg reduction rates)	Observed and reported side effects	References
Uganda	*S. mansoni*	At baseline, a total of 363 pre-school children (≤5 years old) were examined and treated with PZQ. The prevalence of intestinal schistosomiasis was 44.3% (Geometric mean 5.72 epg) in children from Lake Albert and 16% (geometric mean 0.79 epg) for those from Lake Victoria. The intensity of infections for children from Lake Albert were as follows, light intensity of infection (1-100 epg) was 24.4%, moderate intensity (101-400 epg), 11.5% and heavy intensity was (>400 epg) was 8.4%. For the children from Lake Victoria, 12.1% had light intensity, 2.6% had moderate intensity and 1.3% had heavy intensity. At 40 mg/kg, PZQ has had a cure rates of 100% among children detect with patent *S. mansoni* eggs, decreased from 16% to 3.1% after 21 days of chemotherapy. Using CCA as diagnostic criteria, praziquantel had cure rates of 65.1% (83 children positive at baseline) with population prevalence decreasing from 52.3% to 29.4% after 21 days of chemotherapy.	The observed side effects related to the administration of PZQ included:- choking/coughing (0.1%). After 24 hours of treatment, at lake Albert, 2.6% of the children were reported feeling ill, with abdominal pain (0.9%) and diarrhea (0.8%). In Lake Victoria cohort, after 24 hours of treatment, 5.1% of the children reported complaints of abdominal pain and 16.1% had fatigue. Headache was reported by 3.6%, vomiting (9.4%), diarrhea (10.9%) and urticaria/rash (8.9%). Other reported symptoms were dizziness (10.6%), sleepiness (14.7%), vertigo (13.8%), cramps (11.3%) and nausea (8.8%),	[73]

Country	Species	Efficacy of Praziquantel (PZQ) treatment (cure rates and egg reduction rates)	Observed and reported side effects	References
Cote d'Ivoire	*S. haematobium* and *S. mansoni*	A total of 288 pre-school children aged < 6 years were recruited into the study. 160 children had complete data. The prevalence of *S. mansoni* based on Kato Katz technique was 21.9% and based on CCA was 80%. The geometric mean infection intensity was 1.2 epg. At baseline, 65.7% had light infection (1-99 epg), 25.7% had moderate infection (100-399 epg) and 8.6% had heavy infection (≥400 epg).	Of the 234 treated children, 18.37% (43/234) reported to have adverse effects. Of these children, 27.9% were co-infected with *S. mansoni* and *S. haematobium* and 39.5% had *S. mansoni* alone and the remaining 32.6% had no infection. - Within 4 hours after treatment, the following adverse effects were recorded in 32 (74.4%) children:- abdominal pain, diarrhea, nausea, vomiting, dizziness, fever, fatigue, body inflammation and headache. - Some of the children reported combination of adverse effects:- (abdominal pain + diarrhea), (vomiting + nausea) and (fever + dizziness). - 24 hours post-treatment 25.6% of the children reported adverse effects including:- diarrhea, abdominal pain, fatigue, face and body inflammation, dizziness and headache.	[41]
		With regard to *S. haematobium,* the prevalence was 11.2% and geometric mean infection intensity was 1 egg/10 ml of urine. At baseline, 94.4% had light infection (1-49 eggs/10 ml of urine) and 5.5% had heavy infections (≥ 50 eggs/10 ml of urine).		
		Almost 6.9% of the children were co-infected with *S. mansoni* and *S. haematobium.*		
		Using Kato Katz diagnostic technique, three weeks after PZQ treatment (40 mg/kg BWT), the *S. mansoni* prevalence dropped from 21.9% to 2.5% and the cure rate was 88.6% and the Egg reduction rate was 96.7% (from 1.2 epg to 0.04 epg). Based on the CCA results, the cure rates was 38.3%.		
		With regards to *S. haematobium*, the cure rates were 88.9% (decreased from 11.2% to 1.3%). The egg reduction rate was 98% (decreased from 1 eggs/10 ml of urine to 0.02 eggs/10 ml of urine.		

Table 2. (Continued)

Country	Species	Efficacy of Praziquantel (PZQ) treatment (cure rates and egg reduction rates)	Observed and reported side effects	References
Zimbabwe	*S. haematobium*	A total of 100 children aged 1-5 years were recruited. The overall prevalence of *S. haematobium* was 21% with children aged 4-5 years having a prevalence of 25%. The overall mean infection intensity was 14.6 eggs/10 ml of urine and maximum intensity of infection was 458 eggs/10 ml of urine. The mean infection intensity for PZQ treated group at baseline was 9.9 eggs/10 ml of urine and untreated group was 26.8 eggs/10 ml of urine. In 72 children treated with PZQ (40 mg/kg), infection intensity declined from a mean of 9.9 eggs/10 mls of urine, giving egg reduction rate of 99%. The prevalence of *S. haematobium* in treated group, declined from 18% to 1.4%, giving cure rates of 92%.	The adverse effects reported within 24 hours of treatment were diarrhoea (3 children), lethargy (2 children), inflammation of the body and face (1 child) and loss of appetite (1 child).	[44]
Uganda	*S. mansoni*	A total of 979 children were recruited aged 5-93 months. The prevalence of egg-patent was 37.7%, with geometric mean of 5.99 epg, arithmetic mean was 171.2 epg and maximum intensity of 7284 epg. The prevalence of heavy intensity of infection (>399 epg) was 8.9%. Prevalence of urine-CCA positive individuals was 57.1%.	Adverse effects reported were dizziness, sleepiness, fatigue, cramps, nausea, sweating, urticaria, diarrhea, abdominal pain and night fevers.	[65]

Country	Species	Efficacy of Praziquantel (PZQ) treatment (cure rates and egg reduction rates)	Observed and reported side effects	References
Uganda	*S. mansoni*	- The PZQ cure rates in the treatment-naïve children was 77.6% and the egg reduction rate was 92.1% for 1st follow-up and 99.1% in 2nd follow-up. The maximum observed intensity decreased from 7284 epg to 1524 epg, with the arithmetic mean decreasing from 394 epg to 31 epg and geometric mean decreased from 108 epg to 1 epg. - For the previous treated children, the cure rate was 41.7%, egg reduction rate at first follow-up was 72.8% and 2nd follow-up was 92.2%. The maximum intensity of infection decreased from 3906 epg to 3228 epg, with arithmetic mean decreasing from 290 epg to 79 epg. Geometric mean decreased from 102 epg to 8 epg. - Based on CCA results, praziquantel efficacy was 32.3% in naïve-treated group and 20.7% in previous treated group.	Adverse effects reported were dizziness, sleepiness, fatigue, cramps, nausea, sweating, urticaria, diarrhea, abdominal pain and night fevers.	[65]
		A total of 596 children aged 1-4 years were recruited in the study. The overall prevalence of *S. mansoni* was 21.8% with 19.2% of the children having heavy infection (≥400 epg), 20.8% having moderate infection (100-399 epg) and 60% had light infection intensity (1-99 epg). The geometrical mean intensity was 84.6 epg (maximum intensity of 3612 epg) with children aged 4 years recording highest geometric mean intensity of infection (111.5 epg).	Reported adverse effects reported 15 minutes after treatment and 24 hours after treatment, included:- diarrhea, abdominal pain, skin rashes and vomiting.	[48]

Table 2. (Continued)

Country	Species	Efficacy of Praziquantel (PZQ) treatment (cure rates and egg reduction rates)	Observed and reported side effects	References
Uganda	*S. mansoni*	- Treatment groups: The geometric mean of the treatment and control groups were 52.4 epg and 62.4 epg before treatment.	NB: The authors reported only the acceptability and safety of the drugs and no results on efficacy of PZQ.	[48]
Mali	*S. haematobium*	A total of 338 preschool children aged 1-4 years were examined. The overall prevalence was 51.2% (173/338) with no sex differences. Infected children were treated using PZQ (40 mg/kg).	Common side effects reported after 24 hours and 21 days of treatment were:- dizziness, abdominal pain, nausea, diarrhoea, vomiting, headache, sleepiness, fatigue, lower back pain and urticaria/rash.	[56]
Zimbabwe	*S. haematobium*	A total of 595 pre-school children aged ≤6 years were included. The overall prevalence before treatment was 51.8% and was reduced to 7% after treatment. The mean intensity of infection was 18 eggs/10 ml of urine before treatment and decreased to <4 eggs/ 10 ml of urine after two months and 9 eggs/10 ml of urine after 9 months.	Authors did not report/assess side effects of the drug.	[66]

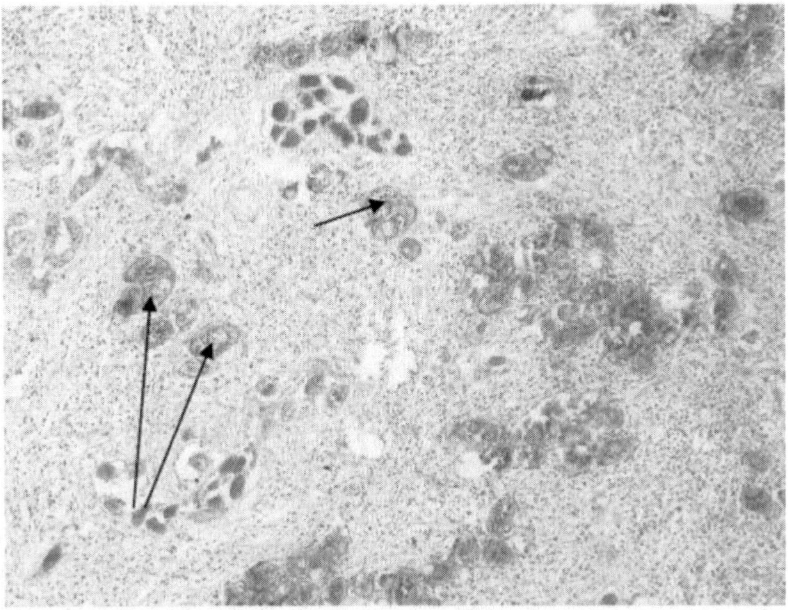

Courtesy of Mazigo HD.

Figure 5. Arrows showing eggs of *S. mansoni* (with lateral spine) in the sub-mucosa and mucosa of the ileum and caecum of a 7 year-old Tanzanian boy presenting with intestinal obstructions in a referral hospital in North-Western Tanzania.

Furthermore, the development of the praziquantel dosing pole, which includes new height intervals (60-84 cm for one-half tablet and 84-99 cm for the three-quarters of one tablet) for smaller children, is a step forward towards the inclusion of the pre-school children in community mass drug administration (Figure 6) [46, 73, 127, 128].

Challenges still remain for the diagnosis and treatment in large-scale control programs. They include: the variation in sensitivity of the diagnostic techniques; the lack of user-friendly praziquantel tablets with marks allowing an easy division into four quarters (in particular when treating children weighing 7.5-11.25 kg); the variation in the efficacy of crushed tablets versus a syrup formulation of praziquantel; the lengthy process of crushing praziquantel tablets [127, 128]. The development of a pediatric formulation of praziquantel, for example flavoured oral-dispersible tablets or mini-tablets, which are easier to administer to a child, is urgently required. In addition, co-infection of schistosomiasis with other co-endemic diseases such as malaria, soil-transmitted helminths and HIV-1 presents another public health challenge for this particular age group.

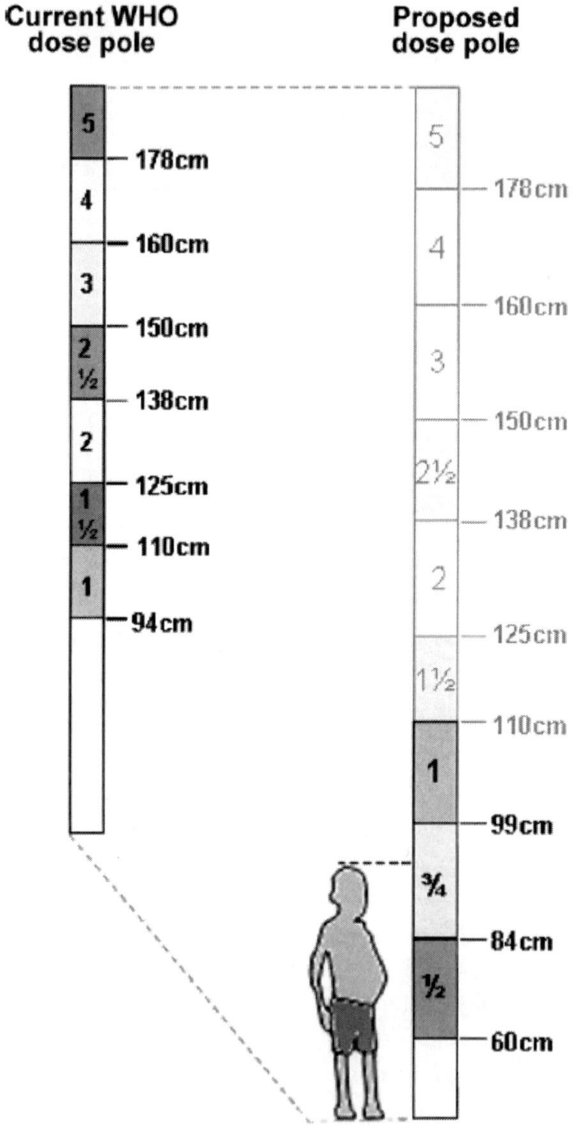

Figure 6. Pictorial representation of the current WHO dose pole for administration of Praziquantel (PZQ) tablets (at 600 mg each) (left) [129] and the proposed dose pole (right) with two new height thresholds added to allow for treatment of preschool children (≤6 year olds): 60–84 cm for one-half and 84–99 cm for three-quarters PZQ tablet [127, 128]. The illustrated child needs three-quarters of one tablet. Additionally, the WHO pole's single tablet lower limit has been amended from 94 cm to 99 cm [127, 128].

There is a need for further recommendations for integrating the control of neglected tropical diseases in programs targeting malaria and HIV-1 in this age group.

References

[1] Ross, A. G. P., Bartley, P. B., Sleigh, A. C., Olds, R., Li, Y., Williams, G. M., McManus, D. P. Schistosomiasis. *N. Engl. J. Med.*, 2002, 346: 1212-1220.

[2] Gryseels, B., Polman, K., Clerinx, J., Kesterns, L. Human schistosomiasis. *Lancet* 2006, 368, 1106-1118.

[3] Pfister, E. Schistosomiasis (Bilharziasis) *Archive Gesch Medicine,* 1912, 6: 12-20.

[4] Ruffer, S. M. A. The presence of ova in mummies and Canopic jar of mummified viscera. *Br. Med. J.,* 1910, 1: 16-25.

[5] Eltawil, K. M., Plassmann, M. Theodor Maximillian Bilharz (1825-1862): The discoverer of Schistosomiasis. *Int. J. Parasitol. Res.*, 2011, 1: 17-25.

[6] Cox, F. E. G. C. History of Human Parasitology. *Clin. Microbiol. Rev.*, 2002, 595–612.

[7] Kloos, H. The paleoepidemiology of schistosomiasis in ancient Egypt. *Hum. Ecol. Rev.*, 2002, 1: 14-25.

[8] Kean, B. H. K. E. and Russel, A. J. (ed.). *Tropical medicine and Parasitology: classic investigations.* 1978, Cornell University Press, Ithaca, N.Y.

[9] Manson, P. Report of a case of bilharzia from the West Indies. *BMJ.* 1902, 1894–1895.

[10] Sambon, L. W. New or little known Africa entozoan. *J. Trop. Med. Hyg.* 1907, 10: 117.

[11] Leiper, R. T. Report to the Advisory Committee of the Tropical Diseases Research Fund, Colonial Office London. *Trop. Dis. Bull.*, 1913, 2:195–196.

[12] Meckel von Hemsbach, J. H. Biology of schistosome complexes. *Microgeologie*, Berlin, 1856; 27-31.

[13] Weiland, D. F. Schistosome of the lower mammal. *Human cestodes*, Cambridge 1858; 12: 23-24.

[14] Wright, W. H. Schistosomiasis as a world problem. *Bull. New York Acad. Med.,* 1968, 44: 301-312.

[15] Warren, K. S., Mahmoud, A. A. F., Muruka, J. F., Whittacker, L. R., Ouma, J. H., Arap Siongok, T. K. *Schistosomiasis haematobium* in coast province of Kenya. Relationship between egg output and morbidity. *Am. J. Trop. Med. Hyg.*, 1979, 28: 864-870.

[16] Chitsulo, L., Engels, D., Montresor, A., Savioli, L. The global status of schistosomiasis and its control. *Acta Trop.* 2000, 77: 41-51.

[17] Warren, K. S. Schistosomiasis: Host-Pathogen Biology. *Rev. Inf. Dis.*, 1982, 4: 4.

[18] Doumenge, J. P., Mott, K. E., Reud-Thomas, G. *Atlas of the Global distribution of schistosomiasis: Talence, CEGET-CNRS, Geneva/WHO Publication*. 1987, 233-241.

[19] Jordan, P., Webbe, G., Sturrock, R. *Human schistosomiasis*. Wallingford, England: CAB, 1993.

[20] Mitchell, G. F. Immunopathology of schistosomiasis. *Rev. Med. Microbiol.*, 1990, 101-107.

[21] Jordan, P., Webbe, G. Epidemiology of schistosomiasis, In: *Schistosomiasis, Epidemiology, Treatment and Control*. Heinemann Medical Books, London, 1982, 227-229.

[22] Han, Z. G., Brindley, P. J., Wang, S. Y., Chen, Z. Schistosoma genomics: new perspectives on schistosome biology and host-parasite interaction. *Annu. Rev. Genomics Hum. Genet.* 2009, 10: 211-240.

[23] Ross, A. G. P., Bartley, P. B., Sleigh, A. C., Olds, R., Li, Y., Williams, G. M., McManus, D. P. Schistosomiasis. *N. Engl. J. Med.*, 2002, 346: 1212-1220.

[24] Hotez, P. J. and Kamath, A. Neglected Tropical Diseases in Sub-Saharan Africa: Review of Their Prevalence, Distribution, and Disease Burden. *PLoS Negl. Trop. Dis.*, 2009, 3(8): e412.

[25] Southgate, V. R., Rollinson, D., Tchuem Tchuente, L. A., Hagan, P. Towards control of schistosomiasis in sub-Saharan Africa. *J. Helminth.*, 2005, 79: 181-185.

[26] Van der Werf, M. J., de Vlas, S. J., Brooker, S., Looman, C. W., Nagelkerke, N. J., Habbema, J. D., Engels, D. Quantification of clinical morbidity associated with schistosome infection in sub-Saharan Africa. *Acta Trop.* 2003, 86: 125–139.

[27] Steinmann, P., Keiser, J., Bos, R., Tannel, M., Utzinger, J. Schistosomiasis and water resources development: systematic review, meta-analysis and estimates of people at risk. *Lancet* 2006, 6: 411–425.

[28] Barakat, R., Farghaly, A., El Masry, A. G., El-Sayed, M. K., Hussein, M. H. The epidemiology of schistosomiasis in Egypt: patterns of

Schistosoma mansoni infection and morbidity in Kafr El-Sheikh. *Am. J. Trop. Med. Hyg.*, 2000, 62: 21–27.

[29] King, C. H. Parasites and poverty: the case of schistosomiasis. *Acta Trop.*, 2010, 113: 95–104.

[30] Wynn, T. A., Thompson, R. W., Cheever, A. W., Mentink-Kane, M. M. Immunopathogenesis of schistosomiasis. *Immunol. Rev.* 2004, 201: 156–167.

[31] Barreto, M. L. Geographical and social economic factors relating to the distribution of *S. mansoni* infection in an urban area of north-east Brazil. *Bulletin of World Health Organization* 1991, 93-102.

[32] Huang, Y. and Manderson, L. Schistosomiasis and the social patterning of infection. *Acta Trop.* 1992, 51, 175-194.

[33] Marcal Junior, O., Hotta, L. K., Patucci, R. M. J., Glasser, C. M., Dias, L. C. S. Schistosomiasis mansoni in an area of low transmission, II. Risk factors for infection. *Rev. Inst. Med. Trop. Sao Paulo,* 1993, 35: 331-335.

[34] Fulford, A. J., Ouma, J. H., Kariuki, H. C., Thiongo, E. W., Klumpp, R., Kloos, H., Butterworth, A. E. Water contact observations in Kenyan communities' endemic for schistosomiasis; methodology and patterns of behaviour. *Parasitol.*, 1996, 113: 223-241.

[35] Modha, J., Redman, C. A., Thornhill, J., Kusel, J. R. Schistosomes; Unanswered questions on the Basic Biology of the host-parasite Relationship. *Parasitol. Today*, 1998, 14: 396-401.

[36] Woolhouse, M. E. J. Patterns in parasite epidemiology; the peak shift. *Parasitol. Today* 1998, 14: 428-34.

[37] Malenganisho, W. L., Magnussen, P., Friis, H., Siza, J., Kaatano, G., Temu, M., Vennervald, B. J. *Schistosoma mansoni* morbidity among adults in two villages along Lake Victoria shores in Mwanza District, Tanzania. *Trans. R Soc. Trop. Med. Hyg.*, 2008, 102: 532-541.

[38] Kabetereine, N. B., Vennervald, B. J., Ouma, J. H., Kemijumbi, J., Butterworth, A. E., Dunne, D. W., Fulford, A. J. C. Adult resistance to schistosomiasis mansoni: age-dependence of re-infection remains in communities with diverse exposure patterns. *Parasitol.* 1999, 118: 101–105.

[39] Lwambo, N. J. S., Siza, J. E., Brooker, S., Bundy, D. A. P., Guyatt, H. Patterns of concurrent hookworm infection and schistosomiasis in schoolchildren in Tanzania. *Trans. R Soc. Trop. Med. Hyg.* 1999, 93: 497-502.

[40] Stothard, J. R., Sousa-Figueiredo, J. C., Betson, M., Green, H. K., Seto, E. Y. W., Garba, A., Sacko, M., Mutapi, F., van Nery, S., Amin, M. A., Mutumba-Nakalembe, M., Navaratnam, A., Fenwick, A., Kabatereine, N. B., Gabrielli, A. F., Montresor, A. Closing the praziquantel treatment gap: new steps in epidemiological monitoring and control of schistosomiasis in African infants and preschool-aged children. *Parasitol.*, 2011, 138: 1593-1606.

[41] Coulibaly, J. T., N'Gbesso, Y. K., Knopp, S., Keiser, J., N'Goran, E. K., Utzinger, J. Efficacy and Safety of Praziquantel in Preschool-Aged Children in an Area Co-Endemic for *Schistosoma mansoni* and *S. haematobium*. *PLoS Negl. Trop. Dis.*, 2012, 6(12): e1917.

[42] Ekpo, U. F., Oluwole, A. S., Abe, E. M., Etta, H. E., Olamiju, F., Mafiana, C. F. Schistosomiasis in infants and pre-school-aged children in sub-Saharan Africa: implication for control. *Parasitol.*, 2012, 139: 835-41.

[43] Dabo, A., Badawi, H. M., Bary, B., Doumbo, O. K. Urinary schistosomiasis among preschool-aged children in Sahelian rural communities in Mali. *Parasit. Vectors* 2011, 4: 21.

[44] Mutapi, F., Rujeni, N., Bourke, C., Mitchell, K., Appleby, L., Nausch, N., Midzi, N., Mduluza, T. *Schistosoma haematobium* treatment in 1-5 year old children: safety and efficacy of the antihelminthic drug praziquantel. *PLos Negl. Trop. Dis.*, 2011, 5: e1143.

[45] Stothard, J. R., Gabrielli, A. F. Schistosomiasis in African infants and preschool children: to treat or not to treat? *Trends Parasitol.,* 2007, 23: 83-86.

[46] Sthothard, J. R., Sousa-Figueiredo, J. C., Betson, M., Bustinduy, A., Reinhard-Rupp, J. Schistosomiasis in African infants and preschool children: let them now be treated! *Trends Parasitol.,* 2013, 29: 197-205.

[47] World Health Organization. Schistosomiasis and soil-transmitted infections. *54th World Health Assembly, agenda item 13.3 resolution WHA 54.19.*

[48] Namwanje, H., Kabatereine, N. B., Olsen, A. The acceptability and safety of praziquantel alone and in combination with mebendazole in the treatment of Schistosoma mansoni and soil-transmitted helminthiasis in children aged 1-4 years in Uganda. *Parasitol.*, 2011, 138: 1586-1592.

[49] World Health organization. Preventive chemotherapy in Human Helminthiasis. *Coordinated use of anthelminthic drugs in Human Interventions: A Manual for Health Professional and Programme Managers.* World Health Organization, Geneva.

[50] World Health Organization. *Report of a meeting to review the results of studies on the treatment of schistosomiasis in preschool-age children.* Geneva, Switzerland, 13–14 September 2010.

[51] Mafiana, C. F., Ekpo, U. F., Ojo, D. A. Urinary schistosomiasis in preschool children in settlements around Oyan Reservoir in Ogun State, Nigeria: implications for control. *Trop. Med. Int. Health*, 2003, 8: 78-82.

[52] Bosompem, K. M., Bentum, I. A., Otchere, J., Anyan, W. K., Brown, C. A., Osada, Y., Takeo, S., Kojima, S., Ohta, N. Infant schistosomiasis in Ghana: a survey in an irrigation community. *Trop. Med. Intern. Health*, 2004, 9: 917-922.

[53] Opara, K. N., Udoidung, N. I., Ukpong, I. G. Genitourinary schistosomiasis among pre-primary schoolchildren in a rural community within the Cross River Basin, Nigeria. *J. Helminth.*, 2007, 81: 393-397.

[54] Ekpo, U. F., Laja-Deile, A., Oluwole, A. S., Sam-Wobo, S. O., Mafiana, C. F. Urinary schistosomiasis among preschool children in a rural community near Abeokuta, Nigeria. *Parasit. Vectors* 2010, 3: 58.

[55] Garba, A., Barkire, N., Djibo, A., Lamine, M. S., Sofo, B., Gouvras, A. N., Bosque-Oliva, E., Webster, J. P., Stothard, J. R., Utzinger, J., Fenwick, A. Schistosomiasis in infants and preschool-aged children: Infection in a single *Schistosoma haematobium* and a mixed *S. haematobium-S. mansoni* foci of Niger. *Acta Trop.* 2010, 115: 212-219.

[56] Dabo, A., Badawi, H. M., Bary, B., Doumbo, O. K. Urinary schistosomiasis among preschool-aged children in Sahelian rural communities in Mali. *Parasit. Vectors* 2011, 4: 21.

[57] Hodges, M. H., Paye, J., Koroma, M. M., Nyorkor, E. D., Fofonah, I., Zhang, Y. High level of *Schistosoma mansoni* infection in pre-school children in Sierra Leone highlights the need in targeting this age group for praziquantel treatment. *Acta Trop.* 2012, 124: 120-125.

[58] Ekpo, U. F., Oluwole, A. S., Abe, E. M., Etta, H. E., Olamiju, F., Mafiana, C. F. Schistosomiasis in infants and pre-school-aged children in sub-Saharan Africa: implication for control. *Parasitology*, 2012, 139: 835-841.

[59] Odogwu, S. E., Ramamurthy, N. K., Kabatereine, N. B., Kazibwe, F., Tukahebwa, E., Webster, J. P., Fenwick, A., Stothard, J. R. *Schistosoma mansoni* in infants (aged < 3 years) along the Ugandan shoreline of Lake Victoria. *Ann. Trop. Med. Parasitol.*, 2006, 100: 315-326.

[60] Betson, M., Sousa-Figueiredo, J. C., Rowell, C., Kabatereine, N. B., Stothard, J. R. Intestinal schistosomiasis in mothers and young children

in Uganda: investigation of field-applicable markers of bowel morbidity. *Am. J. Trop. Med. Hyg.* 2010, 83: 1048-1055.

[61] Verani, J. R., Abudho, B., Montgomery, S. P., Mwinzi, P. N., Shane, H. L., Butler, S. E., Karanja, D. M., Secor, W. E. Schistosomiasis among young children in Usoma, Kenya. *Am. J. Trop. Med. Hyg.* 2011, 84: 787-789.

[62] Green, H. K., Sousa-Figueiredo, J. C., Basanez, M. G., Betson, M., Kabatereine, N. B., Fenwick, A., Stothard, J. R. Anaemia in Ugandan preschool-aged children: the relative contribution of intestinal parasites and malaria. *Parasitology* 2011, 138: 1534-1545.

[63] Seto, E. Y. W., Sousa-Figueiredo, J. C., Betson, M., Byalero, C., Kabatereine, N. B., Stothard, J. R., Patterns of intestinal schistosomiasis among mothers and young children from Lake Albert, Uganda: water contact and social networks inferred from wearable global positioning system data loggers. *Geospatial. Health* 2012, 7: 1-13.

[64] Stothard, J. R., Sousa-Figuereido, J. C., Betson, M., Adriko, M., Arinaitwe, M., Rowell, C., Besiyge, F., Kabatereine, N. B. *Schistosoma mansoni* infections in young children: When are schistosome antigens in urine, eggs in stool and antibodies to egg first detectable? *PLOS Negl. Trop. Dis.* 2011, 5: e938.

[65] Sousa-Figueiredo, J. C., Betson, M., Atuhaire, A., Arinaitwe, M., Navaratnam, A. M. D., Kabatereine, N. B., Bickle, Q., Stothard, J. R. Performance and Safety of Praziquantel for Treatment of Intestinal Schistosomiasis in Infants and Preschool Children. *PLos Negl. Trop. Dis.*, 2012, 6:10:e1864.

[66] Mduluza, T., Ndhlovu, P. D., Madziwa, T. M., Midzi, N., Zinyama, R., Turner, C. M., Chandiwana, S. K., Nyazema, N., Hagan, P. The impact of repeated treatment with praziquantel of schistosomiasis in children under six years of age living in an endemic area for *Schistosoma haematobium* infection. *Mem. Inst. Oswaldo Cruz*, 2001, 96: 157-164.

[67] Forsyth, D. M. and MacDonald, G. Urological complications of endemic schistosomiasis in school-children. Part 1. Usagara school. *Trans. R Soc. Trop. Med. Hyg.*, 1965, 59: 171-178.

[68] Forsyth, D. M. and Bradley, D. J. The consequences of Bilhaziasis. Medical and Public health importance in North-west Tanzania. *Bulletin WHO*. 1966, 34: 715-735.

[69] Hatz, C., Savioli, L., Mayombana, C., Dhunputh, J., Kisumku, U. M., Tanner, M. Measurement of schistosomiasis-related morbidity at

community level in areas of different endemicity. *Bulletin WHO* 1990, 66: 777-787.

[70] Hatz, C., Mayombana, C., de Savigny, D., MacPherson, C. N., Koella, J. C., Degrémont, A., Tanner, M. Ultrasound scanning for detecting morbidity due to *Schistosoma haematobium* and its resolution following treatment with different doses of praziquantel. *Trans. R Soc. Trop. Med. Hyg*. 1990, 84: 84-88.

[71] King, C. H., Dangerfield-Cha, M. The unacknowledged impact of chronic schistosomiasis. *Chronic Ill.* 2008, 4: 65-79.

[72] Webster, J. P., Koukounari, A., Lamberton, P. H., Stothard, J. R., Fenwick, A. Evaluation and application of potential schistosome-associated morbidity markers within large-scale mass chemotherapy programmes. *Parasitology* 2009, 136: 1789-1799.

[73] Sousa-Figueiredo, J. C., Pleasant, J., Day, M., Betson, M., Rollinson, D., Montresor, A., Kazibwe, F., Kabatereine, N. B., Stothard, J. R. Treatment of intestinal schistosomiasis in Ugandan preschool children: best diagnosis, treatment efficacy and side-effects, and an extended praziquantel dosing pole. *Int. Health*, 2010, 2: 103-113.

[74] Boisier, P., Serieye, J., Ravaoalimalala, V. E., Roux, J., Esterre, P.: Ultrasonographical assessment of morbidity in schistosomiasis mansoni in Madagascar: a community-based study in a rural population. *Trans. R Soc. Trop. Med. Hyg.*, 1995, 89: 208–212.

[75] Pitkanen, Y. T., Peltonen, M., Lahdevirta, J., Meri, S., Evengard, B., Linder, E. Acute schistosomiasis mansoni in Finnish hunters visiting Africa: need for appropriate diagnostic serology. *Scand. J. Infect. Dis.*, 1990, 22: 597-600.

[76] Chunge, C. N., Chunge, R. N., Masinde, M. S., Atinga, J. N. An outbreak of acute schistosomiasis following a church retreat to Mwanza, Tanzania, 2008. *J. Trav. Med.*, 2011; 18: 408-410.

[77] Warren, K. S. The immunopathogenesis of schistosomiasis: a multidisciplinary approach. *Trans. R Soc. Trop. Med. Hyg*. 1972, 66: 417-434.

[78] Doherty, F., Moody, A. H., Wright, S. G. Katayama fever: an acute manifestation of schistosomiasis. *BMJ*, 1996, 313: 1071-1072.

[79] Stuiver, P. C. Acute schistosomiasis (Katayama fever). *BMJ*, 1984, 288: 221-222.

[80] Ross, A. G., Vickers, D., Olds, G. R., Shah, S. M., McManus, D. P. Katayama syndrome. *Lancet Inf. Dis.*, 2007, 7: 218-224.

[81] Warren, K. S., Domingo, E. O., Cowan, R. B. Granuloma formation around schistosome eggs as a manifestation of delayed hypersensitivity. *Am. J. Pathol.* 1967, 51: 735–756.

[82] Cheever, A. W., Hoffmann, K. F., Wynn, T. A. Immunopathology of schistosomiasis mansoni in mice and men. *Immunol. Today* 2000, 21: 465–466.

[83] Boros, D. L. and Warren, K. S. Delayed hypersensitivity-type granuloma formation and dermal reaction induced and elicited by a soluble factor isolated from *Schistosoma mansoni* eggs. *J. Exp. Med.*, 1970; 132: 488-507.

[84] Doenhoff, M. J., Pearson, S., Dunne, D. W., Bickle, Q., Lucas, S., Bain, J., Musallam, R., Hassounah, O. Immunological control of hepatotoxicity and parasite egg excretion in Schistosoma mansoni infections: stage specificity of the reactivity of immune serum in T-cell deprived mice. *Trans. R Soc. Trop. Med. Hyg.*, 1981, 75: 41-53.

[85] Vennervald, B. J., Dunne, D. W. Morbidity in schistosomiasis: an update. *Curr. Opin. Infect. Dis.* 2004, 17: 439–447.

[86] Mazigo, H. D., Lwambo, N. J. S., Mkoji, G. M., Laurent, L. M., Kweka, E. J., Waihenya, R. Anaemia and organomegaly associated with parasitic infections among schoolchildren in Sengerema District, north-western Tanzania. *Tanzania J. Health Res.*, 2010, 12 (3).

[87] Kabatereine, N. B., Kemijumbi, J., Ouma, J. H., Kariuki, H. C., Richter, J., Kadzo, H., Madse, H., Butterworth, A. E., Ørnbjerg, N., Vennervald, B. J. Epidemiology and morbidity of *Schistosoma mansoni* infection in a fishing community along Lake Albert in Uganda. *Trans. R Soc. Trop. Med. Hyg.*, 2004, 98: 711–718.

[88] Booth, M., Vennervald, B. J., Kenty, L., Butterworth, A. E., Kariuki, H. C., Kadzo, H., Ireri, E., Amaganga, C., Kimani, G., Mwatha, J. K., Otedo, A., Ouma, J. H., Muchiri, E., Dunne, D. W. Micro-geographical variation in exposure to *Schistosoma mansoni* and malaria, and exacerbation of splenomegaly in Kenyan school-aged children. *BMC Infect. Dis.* 2004, 17: 13.

[89] Dunne, D. W., Pearce, E. J. Immunology of hepatosplenic schistosomiasis mansoni: a human perspective. *Microbes Infect.*, 1999, 1: 553–560.

[90] Gryseels, B., Polderman, A. M. The morbidity of schistosomiasis mansoni in Maniema (Zaire). *Trans. R Soc. Trop. Med. Hyg.* 1987, 81: 202–209.

[91] Kardorff, R., Gabone, R. M., Mugashe, C., Obiga, D., Ramarokoto, C. E., Mahlert, C., Spannbrucker, N., Lang, A., Gunzler, V., Gryseels, B., Ehrich, J. H. H., Doehring, E. *Schistosoma mansoni*-related morbidity on Ukerewe Island, Tanzania: clinical, ultrasonographical and biochemical parameters. *Trop. Med. Int. Health*, 1997, 2: 230–239.

[92] Mazigo, H. D., Chandika, A. B., Zinga, M., Heukelbach, J., Rambau, P. Intestinal schistosomiasis associated with intussusception: a case report. *Tanzania J. Health Res.*, 2011, 13(2).

[93] King, C. H. Disease in schistosomiasis haematobia. In: *Schistosomiasis*. Edited by Mahmoud, A. A. F. London: Imperial College Press; 2001, 265–295.

[94] Hatz, C. F., Vennervald, B. J., Nkulila, T., Vounatsou, P., Kombe, Y., Mayombana, C., Mshinda, H., Tanner, M. Evolution of *Schistosoma haematobium*-related pathology over 24 months after treatment with praziquantel among school children in Southern-eastern Tanzania. *Am. J. Trop. Med. Hyg.*, 1998, 59: 775–781.

[95] Brito, L. L., Barreto, M. L., Silva Rde, C., Assis, A. M., Reis, M. G., Parraga, I. M., Blanton, R. E. Moderate- and low-intensity co-infections by intestinal helminths and *Schistosoma mansoni*, dietary iron intake, and anemia in Brazilian children. *Am. J. Trop. Med. Hyg.*, 2006; 75: 939-944.

[96] Koukounari, A., Fenwick, A., Whawell, S., Kabatereine, N. B., Kazibwe, F., Tukahebwa, E. M., Stothard, J. R., Donnelly, C. A., Webster, J. P. Morbidity indicators of Schistosoma mansoni: relationship between infection and anemia in Ugandan schoolchildren before and after praziquantel and albendazole chemotherapy. *Am. J. Trop. Med. Hyg.* 2006, 75: 278-286.

[97] Koukounari, A., Gabrielli, A. F., Toure, S., Bosque-Oliva, E., Zhang, Y., Sellin, B., Donnelly, C. A., Fenwick, A., Webster, J. P. *Schistosoma haematobium* infection and morbidity before and after large-scale administration of praziquantel in Burkina Faso. *J. Infect. Dis.*, 2007, 196: 659-669.

[98] Green, H. K., Sousa-Figueiredo, J. C., Basanez, M. G., Betson, M., Kabatereine, N. B., Fenwick, A., Stothard, J. R. Anaemia in Ugandan preschool-aged children: the relative contribution of intestinal parasites and malaria. *Parasitology*, 2011, 138: 1534-1545.

[99] Sturrock, R. F., Kariuki, H. C., Thiongo, F. W., Gachare, J. W., Omondi, B. G., Ouma, J. H., Mbugua, G., Butterworth, A. E. *Schistosomiasis mansoni* in Kenya: relationship between infection and anaemia in

schoolchildren at the community level. *Trans. R Soc. Trop. Med. Hyg.* 1996, 90: 48-54.

[100] Prual, A., Daouda, H., Develoux, M., Sellin, B., Galan, P., Hercberg, S. Consequences of *Schistosoma haematobium* infection on the iron status of schoolchildren in Niger. *Am. J. Trop. Med. Hyg.* 1992, 47: 291-297.

[101] Partnership for Child: Development Heavy schistosomiasis associated with poor short-term memory and slower reaction times in Tanzanian schoolchildren. *Trop. Med. Int. Health* 2002, 7: 104–117.

[102] Stoltzfus, R. J., Albanico, M., Tielsch, J. M., Chwaya, H. M., Savioli, L. Linear Growth Retardation in Zanzibarian School Children. *J. Nutrition* 1997, 27: 1099–1105.

[103] Dickson, R., Awasthi, S., Williamson, P., Demellweek, C., Garner, P. (2000) Effects of treatment for intestinal helminth infection on growth and cognitive performance in children: systematic review of randomised trials. *Brit. Med. J.*, 2000, 320: 1697–1701.

[104] Stephenson, L. S., Latham, M. C., Kurz, K. M., Kinoti, S. N. Single dose Metrifonate or praziquantel treatment in Kenyan children. II. Effects on growth in relation to Schistosoma haematobium and hookworm egg counts. *Am. J. Trop. Med. Hyg.*, 1989, 41: 445–453.

[105] Tohon, Z. B., Mainassara, H. B., Garba, A., Mahamane, A. E., Bosque-Oliva, E., Maman-Laminou, I., Duchemin, J. B., Chanteau, S., Boisier, P. Controlling Schistosomiasis: Significant Decrease of Anaemia Prevalence One Year after a Single Dose of Praziquantel in Nigerian Schoolchildren. *PLoS Negl. Trop. Dis.*, 2008, 2: e241.

[106] World Health Organization. Guidelines for the evaluation of soil-transmitted helminthiasis and schistosomiasis at community level. *A guide for managers of control programmes, 1998. WHO/CTD/SIP/98.1.*

[107] Navaratnam, A. M., Mutumba-Nakalembe, M. J., Stothard, J. R., Kabetereine, N. B., Fenwick, A., Sousa-Figueiredo, J. C. Notes on the use of urine-CCA dipsticks for detection of intestinal schistosomiasis in preschool children. *Trans. R Soc. Trop. Med. Hyg.*, 2012, 106: 619-622.

[108] Stothard, J. R., Kabatereine, N. B., Tukahebwa, E. M., Kazibwe, F., Rollinson, D., Mathieson, W., Webster, J. P., Fenwick, A. Use of circulating cathodic antigen (CCA) dipsticks for detection of intestinal and urinary schistosomiasis. *Acta Trop.*, 2006, 97: 219-228.

[109] Sousa-Figueiredo, J. C., Betson, M., Kabatereine, N. B., Stothard, J. R. The urine circulating cathodic antigen (CCA) dipstick: a valid substitute for microscopy for mapping and point-of-care diagnosis of intestinal schistosomiasis. *PLoS Negl. Trop. Dis.*, 2013, 7:1:e2008.

[110] Doenhoff, M., Musallam, R., Bain, J., McGregor, A. Studies on the host-parasite relationship in Schistosoma mansoni-infected mice: the immunological dependence of parasite egg excretion. *Immunology*, 1978, 35: 771-778.

[111] Coulibaly, J. T., N'Goran, E. K., Utzinger, J., Doenhoff, M. J., Dawson, E. M. A new rapid diagnostic test for detection of anti-*Schistosoma mansoni* and anti-*Schistosoma haematobium* antibodies. *Parasit. Vectors* 2013, 6: 29.

[112] Ashton, R. A., Stewart, B. T., Petty, N., Lado, M., Finn, T., Brooker, S., Kolaczinski, J. H. Accuracy of circulating cathodic antigen tests for rapid mapping of *Schistosoma mansoni* and *S. haematobium* infections in Southern Sudan. *Trop. Med. Int. Health*, 2011, 16: 1099-1103.

[113] Ten Hove, R. J., Verweij, J. J., Vereecken, K., Polman, K., Dieye, L., van Lieshout, L. Multiplex real-time PCR for the detection and quantification of *Schistosoma mansoni* and *S. haematobium* infection in stool samples collected in northern Senegal. *Trans. R Soc. Trop. Med. Hyg.*, 2008, 102: 179-185.

[114] Obeng, B. B., Aryeetey, Y. A., de Dood, C. J., Amoah, A. S., Larbi, I. A., Deelder, A. M., Yazdanbakhsh, M., Hartgers, F. C., Boakye, D. A., Verweij, J. J., van Dam, G. J., van Lieshout, L. Application of a circulating-cathodic-antigen (CCA) strip test and real-time PCR, in comparison with microscopy, for the detection of *Schistosoma haematobium* in urine samples from Ghana. *Ann. Trop. Med. Parasitol.*, 2008, 102: 625-633.

[115] Pontes, L. A., Oliveira, M. C., Katz, N., Dias-Neto, E., Rabello, A. Comparison of a polymerase chain reaction and the Kato-Katz technique for diagnosing infection with *Schistosoma mansoni*. *Am. J. Trop. Med. Hyg.*, 2003, 68: 652-656.

[116] Lwambo, N. J. S., Savioli, L., Kisumku, U. M., Alawi, K. S., Bundy, D. A. P. Control of *Schistosoma haematobium* morbidity on Pemba Island: validity and efficiency of indirect screening tests. *Bull. WHO*, 1997, 75 (3): 247-252.

[117] Sousa-Figueiredo, J. C., Basanez, M. G., Khamis, I. S., Garba, A., Rollinson, D., Stothard, J. R. Measuring morbidity associated with urinary schistosomiasis: assessing levels of excreted urine albumin and urinary tract pathologies. *PLOS Negl. Trop. Dis.*, 2009, 3: e526.

[118] Lengeler, C., Makwala, J., Ngimbi, D., Utzinger, J. Simple school questionnaires can map both *Schistosoma mansoni* and *Schistosoma*

haematobium in the Democratic Republic of Congo. *Acta Trop.*, 2000, 74: 77-87.

[119] Lengeler, C., Utzinger, J., Tanner, M. Screening for schistosomiasis with questionnaires. *Trends Parasitol.*, 2002, 18: 375-377.

[120] World Health Organization: Schistosomiasis and soil-transmitted infections. *54th World Health Assembly, agenda item 13.3 resolution WHA 54.19.*

[121] Midzi, N., Sangweme, D., Zinyowera, S., Mapingure, M. P., Brouwer, K. C., Kumar, N., Mutapi, F., Woelk, G., Mduluza, T. Efficacy and side effects of praziquantel treatment against *Schistosoma haematobium* infection among primary school children in Zimbabwe. *Trans. R Soc. Trop. Med. Hyg.*, 2008, 102: 759-766.

[122] Berhe, N., Gundersen, S. G., Abebe, F., Birrie, H., Medhin, G., Gemetchu, T. Praziquantel side effects and efficacy related to *Schistosoma mansoni* egg loads and morbidity in primary school children in north-east Ethiopia. *Acta Trop.* 1999, 72: 53-63.

[123] King, C. H. Long-term outcomes of school-based treatments for control of urinary schistosomiasis: A review of experience in Coast Province, Kenya. *Mem. Inst. Oswaldo Cruz*, 2006, 101: 299-306.

[124] Mitchell, K. M., Mutapi, F., Savill, N. J., Woolhouse, M. E. Protective immunity to *Schistosoma haematobium* infection is primarily an anti-fecundity response stimulated by the death of adult worms. *Proc. Natl. Acad. Sci. US*, 2012, 109: 13347-1352.

[125] Frenzel, K., Grigull, L., Odongo-Aginya, E., Ndugwa, C. M., Loroni-Lakwo, T., Schweigmann, U., Vester, U., Spannbrucker, N., Doehring, E. Evidence for a long-term effect of a single dose of praziquantel on *Schistosoma mansoni*-induced hepatosplenic lesions in northern Uganda. *Am. J. Med. Hyg.*, 1999, 60: 927-931.

[126] Kabatereine, N. B., Brooker, S., Koukonauri, A., Kazibwe, F., Tukahebwa, E. M., Fleming, F. M., Zhang, Y., Webster, J. P., Stothard, J. R., Fenwick, A. Impact of a national control helminth control programme on infection and morbidity in Ugandan schoolchildren. *Bull. WHO* 2007, 85: 91-99.

[127] Sousa-Figueiredo, J. C., Day, M., Betson, M., Kabatereine, N. B., Stothard, J. R. An inclusive dose pole for treatment of schistosomiasis in infants and preschool children with praziquantel. *Trans. R Soc. Trop. Med. Hyg.*, 2010, 104: 740-742.

[128] Sousa-Figueiredo, J. C., Betson, M., Stothard, J. R. Treatment of schistosomiasis in African infants and preschool-aged children:

downward extension and biometric optimization of the current praziquantel dose pole. *Int. Health*, 2012, 4: 95-102.
[129] Montresor, A., Odermatt, P., Muth, S. The WHO dose pole for the administration of praziquantel is also accurate in non-African populations. *Trans. R Soc. Trop. Med. Hyg.*, 2005, 99: 78–81.

In: Schistosomiasis
Editor: Adriana Erica Miele
ISBN: 978-1-63117-186-4

Chapter 7

The Pathologic Spectrum of Incidental Biopsy-Diagnosed Schistosomiasis in the Limpopo Province, South Africa, with Special Emphasis on Female Urogenital Schistosomiasis

Louis-Jacques van Bogaert*
National Health Laboratory Service, Polokwane/Mankweng Hospital Complex and the University of Limpopo, Limpopo, South Africa

Abstract

Schistosomiasis, the second most common neglected tropical disease, is multifaceted. It is a public health condition intimately dependent on its prevention through water sanitation and preventive chemotherapy in school children. Schistosome infection may affect any part of the body. The pathology it causes is complex and complicated by the possible interaction with carcinogens and other infectious agents. For mainly social and environmental factors, children and adult females are more affected than adult males. The Limpopo Province of South Africa is a

---

* Corresponding Author address: National Health Laboratory Service, Polokwane Hospital, Hospital street, Polokwane, Limpopo, South Africa; Email: louis.vanBogaert@nhls.ac.za.

region of schistosome, human immunodeficiency virus (HIV), and human papilloma virus (HPV) related cervical cancer endemicity. No organized fluke prevention programme is in place.

We studied a series of 672 consecutive cases of biopsy-diagnosed schistosomiasis. The female/male ratio was 3.7/1.0. The HIV female/male ratio was 55.0/1.0.

S. mansoni was identified in 4.9% of the cases; 68.8% of them were cases of urogenital schistosomiasis. Höppli granulomas were diagnosed in 10.0% of all cases. Invasive cancer, mainly cervical and bladder cancer, was associated in 12.1% of the cases.

This illustrates the high burden of disease on women's reproductive health in the absence of preventive measures. It also highlights the importance of school preventive programs, as, among others, a potential prophylaxis against all sexually transmitted infections, especially HIV.

Keywords: Urinary schistosomiasis, urogenital pathologies, co-infections with sexually-transmitted diseases, women fertility, cancer onset

Introduction

Schistosome infection affects more than 200 million people worldwide. About 85% of cases occur in Africa [1]. According to the latest WHO report, only 9.8% of those in need of treatment are actually treated [2]. This is one of the main reasons why schistosomiasis is listed among the Neglected Tropical Diseases (NTD) [3-5]. Urine- or feces-contaminated water is the source of infection; therefore, water sanitation is the mainstay of prevention. For socio-cultural reasons, children and women are the main victims [6]. In the short to median term, annual treatment for school-aged children in areas of high endemicity is essential to prevent the morbidity resulting from anemia, stunted growth, and learning disability. In the long term, it would also limit adult schistosome-related morbidity and mortality [7].

More recently, it has been suggested that urogenital schistosomiasis (UGS), and sexually transmitted infections (STI), disrupt the integrity of the genital mucosa. Any breach in the genital mucosa is potentially an entry or exit portal of STI. The rationale is that prevention of schistosomiasis, especially in school-girls, would prevent UGS at a later age, and the potential STIs, including human immunodeficiency virus (HIV) and the ensuing acquired immuno deficiency syndrome (AIDS) [5, 8-10].

However, at present, preventive measures in terms of water sanitation and school programmes are poorly implemented, especially in sub-Saharan Africa

[11-12]. In South Africa, there is no national program for the control of schistosomiasis in spite of the common occurrence of the infection in many parts of the country [13]. Adding to the problem is the fact that praziquantel kills the adult schistosomes but leaves the ova unscathed. Embryonated ova (containing miracidia) induce a granulomatous tissue reaction first described by Höppli [14]. This corresponds to the so-called "grainy sandy patches" and "homogeneous yellow sandy patches" visible on urogenital mucosa [15-18]. They constitute breaches in the urogenital mucosa. Later on the eggs become calcified and surrounded by connective scar tissue. Praziquantel has no effect on the ova embedded in the tissues. Hence, the importance of early praziquantel treatment before the eggs are deposited in the tissues [10].

A large amount of work has and is still done and published on the immunobiology and benefits of school prevention of schistosomiasis. Relatively little is known on the anatomical distribution and histopathological types of schistosome related lesions. We present a series of 672 consecutive cases of incidentally biopsy-diagnosed schistosomiasis in the Limpopo Province of South Africa. We are well aware that cross-sectional studies allow determination of association rather than a cause-effect relationship. However, the design of prospective studies in this area would be ethically problematic and very complex [1]. The information provided by cross-sectional studies should help public authorities to implement the adequate preventive strategies [13].

Methods

1. Background

Schistosomiasis is endemic in the eastern provinces of South Africa: Kwa-Zulu Natal, Mpumalanga, Limpopo, and Eastern Cape. The Limpopo Province is the most northern province of South Africa. It is bordered from East to West by Mozambique, Zimbabwe, and Botswana. The population is estimated at 5.8 million, or 11.3% of the South African population. The prevalence of HIV is 18.5% [19]. It is estimated that 4.5 to 5.3 million, e.g., approximately 10% of the total South African population is infected by schistosomes and that 2.5 million require preventive chemotherapy [10, 20]. It is estimated that 1 to 2 million South African women suffer from female genital schistosomiasis [10].

2. Clinical and Pathological Data

The National Health Laboratory Service (NHLS) renders services to 37 public hospitals in the Limpopo Province. All histological and cytological specimens are centralized at and handled by the laboratory in the provincial capital Polokwane. On average 10 000 biopsies and 50 000 Pap smears are processed annually. The cases were collected prospectively from 2008 to 2013. None was clinically suspected of schistosomiasis. Most cases were asymptomatic, except those with schistosomal bladder infestation. Fifty five females (10.4%) were HIV-infected; only one male (0.7%) was HIV seropositive.

The diagnosis of schistosomiasis was made on formalin fixed, paraffin embedded, and hematoxylin and eosin stained biopsies. A diagnosis of *Schistosoma haematobium* was made in the presence of a terminal spike, and of *S. mansoni* in the presence of a lateral spike. Embryonated ova were identified by the presence of small dark dots [18- 19]. The diagnosis of Höppli granulomas was made in the presence of large multinucleated histiocytes and an inflammatory infiltrate rich in eosinophils [11].

Results

The geographic distribution of the biopsy-diagnosed cases of schistosomiasis shows that 90.0% were located in North-East quarter of the province bordering Zimbabwe and the Kruger National Park. This area includes the three formerly so-called "Homelands" (or Bantustans in Apartheid terminology) of Venda (bordering Zimbabwe), Gazankulu and Kangwane (bordering the Kruger National Park) (Figure 1).

The Letaba River is the main river in the area; it originates in Venda's Soutpansberg (Saltpan Mountain) and flows down through Gazankulu and Kangwane to Mozambique. The inhabitants usually obtain water for domestic and other uses from springs, wells and streams [13]. Crossed by the tropic of Capricorn, the dividing line between the tropics and southern temperate zones, the province is largely a dry savannah subregion at an altitude between 600 and 900 m above mean sea level. The area bordering the Kruger National Park is also a malaria high-risk area.

The general distribution by gender of Urinary Genital Schistosomiasis (UGS) and non-UGS cases is illustrated in Figure 2. The overall female to male ratio was 3.7:1.0. The prevalence of UGS was 95.0% in females, and

33.0% in males. Table 1 lists the comparative anatomical distribution by gender.

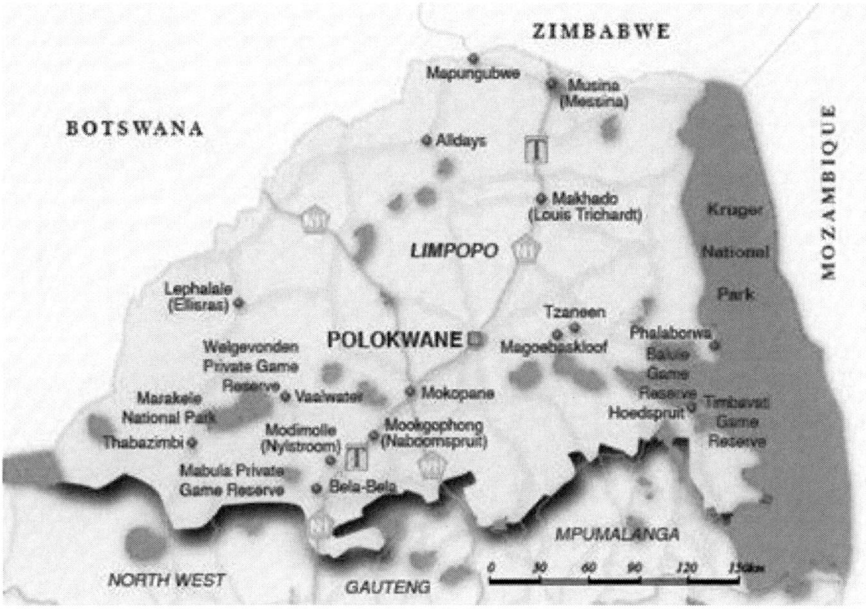

Figure 1. Map of the Limpopo Region, South Africa.

Table 1. Anatomical distribution of schistosomiasis in males and females

Pathology	no. Males (%)	no. Females (%)
Chronic appendicitis	26 (18.2)	10 (1.9)
Acute appendicitis	67 (46.9)	9 (1.7)
Cystitis	28 (19.6)	21 (3.9)
Bladder cancer	7 (4.9)	16 (3.0)
Upper genital	2 (1.4)*	181 (34.3)**
Lower genital	8 (5.6)†	285 (53.9)††
Anus	1 (0.7)	4 (0.7)
Other	4 (2.7)	3 (0.5)
Total	143	529

*Prostate;
** uterine body or adnexae;
†penile shaft, urethra, testis, scrotum;
†† vulva, cervix

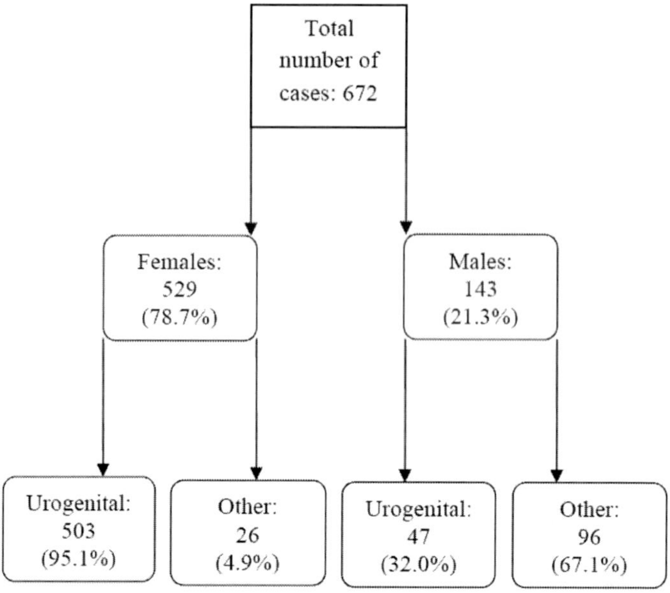

Figure 2. Flow chart of biopsy-diagnosed schistosomiasis.

The anatomical distribution by affected organs in females is shown in Figure 2. A little more than half of the cases involved the uterine cervix. There was a dual localization in 10 instances: ovary and tube (n=1), ovary and cervix (n=3), tube and cervix (n=2), bladder and cervix (n=1), vulva and cervix (n=1), bladder and vulva (n=1), myometrium and pelvic node metastasis of endometrial adenocarcinoma (n=1).

Figure 3 lists the anatomical distribution by affected organs in males. UGS accounted for less than one third, and intestinal pathology (almost exclusively the appendix) for more than two thirds of the localizations.

S. mansoni was identified 33 times (4.9%). Twenty-six were in females: 12 in the cervix, 7 in the fallopian tubes, 3 in the appendix, 2 in the bladder, and one in the vulva and bladder respectively. In males, *S. mansoni* was found 7 times in the appendix, and once in the bladder.

Höppli granulomas were identified in 68 (10.1%) cases. The prevalence of cancer associated schistosome infection was 17.2 % in females (91 invasive cervical carcinomas, 16 bladder, 2 vulvar, and one conjunctival carcinoma). In males, there were 7 bladder cancers (5.3%); of the total 23 bladder cancers, sixteen were of squamous cell type and 7 of urothelial cell type.

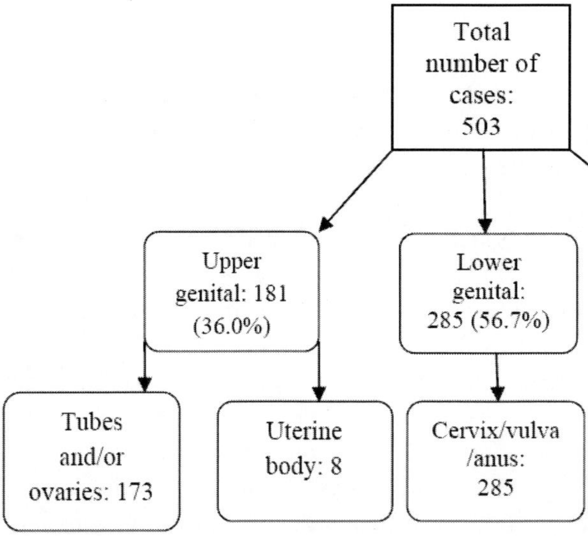

Figure 3. Flow chart of female urogenital schistosomiasis.

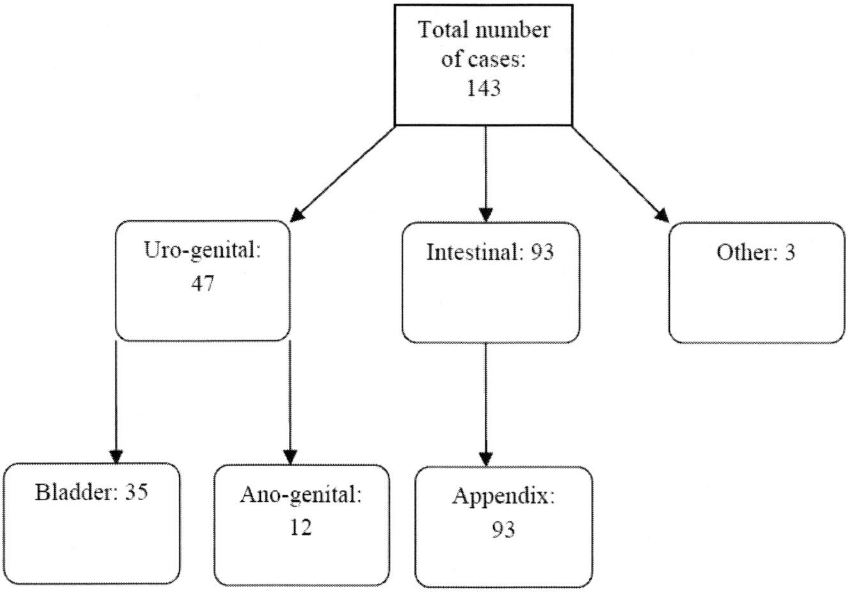

Figure 4. Flow chart of male urogenital schistosomiasis.

Discussion

It is a great pity, not to say a shame, that a preventable tropical disorder that could be contained by simple and cheap means still does not receive the attention it deserves. There is ample knowledge of the source of infection, the life-cycle of schistosomatidae, the way the miracidia penetrate the skin, and their migration inside the body (see also, Chapters 1 and 2 of this book). There is equally ample evidence of the efficacy of preventive chemotherapy in school children. The knowledge is there and yet the implementation is largely lacking.

The great hurdle of water sanitation can be bypassed by preventive chemotherapy, and, possibly by vaccination in the future. The field that still needs research is the immune biology of the infection that would hopefully lead to vaccination. One can only hope that descriptive reports will sensitize public health policy makers and governments to the necessity to pay attention to the infection and implement the required measures [13].

Epidemiological and clinical research on schistosomiasis is usually carried out in relatively strictly controlled settings that may not reflect the reality on the ground because of selection criteria and research protocols. For instance, the study of a relatively small sample of people belonging to a relatively closed community living in a fluke-prone environment is likely to yield an unusual high rate of infestation because of the selected population and the specific research protocol. Our survey shows that in the Limpopo Province only about a quarter of the province is schistosome endemic, while we receive biopsies from the entire province. This illustrates the need for public health programmes to focus more specifically on that part of the province.

Descriptive reports have merits by showing an association between a given pathology and schistosomal infection; however, they cannot prove a causal link. In order to prove a causal relationship between urogenital schistosomal infection and a specific pathology one should withhold praziquantel and follow-up the pathology unfolding. That, of course, would be absolutely unethical. Therefore, in the short and median term, descriptive reports remain the only ethically permissible choice.

Schistosome endemicity is linked to a spectrum of diseases. The association between schistosomes and bladder cancer has been known for decades [23- 25]. A possible link between schistosomiasis and male breast cancer has also been suggested [26- 27]. The morbidity resulting from urogenital schistosomiasis, especially among females, has been widely investigated. It has been suggested that cervical schistosomiasis might act as a co-factor with human papillomavirus (HPV) in cervical carcinogenesis. On the other hand, the postulate that UGS favors a swifter progression of pre-invasive to invasive cervical cancer through the exacerbation of the effects of HPV infection is not supported by any convincing evidence. The reported association of the two conditions is low [17, 28-30]. It appears that it is HPV *per se* that is the necessary carcinogen [28-29, 31-32]. This does not rule out the fact that schistosome-induced mucosal barrier rupture contributes to facilitating HPV transmission.

Finally, according to the same rationale, the possible role of UGS in the transmission of the human immunodeficiency virus (HIV) is currently strongly suspected [1, 3-4, 8, 33-36]. The hypothesis that UGS in both genders might be a significant risk factor for HIV transmission sounds plausible. The inflammatory cells in Höppli granulomas express CD4+ T-cell receptors that are the primary target of HIV to whom they bind. *S. haematobium* infection stimulates the Th2-type immune response, and down-regulates the Th1-type cytotoxic response that is important in the initial control of HIV infection [1]. In addition, *S. haematobium* infections raise the viral load in co-infected subjects [37].

Most studies show that adult schistosomiasis is predominantly affecting women. The most affected part of women's anatomy is the uro-genital system. Therefore, UGS is a threat to women's reproductive health. An early Egyptian study on 88 cases of female UGS reported 74 cases (84.1%) of lower genital localization [38]. A lot of attention has been paid to the naked eye or colposcopically visible so-called "sandy patches" in the female lower genital system, a cause of disruption of the lower genital mucous cutaneous protection [15, 16, 17, 18]. In a series of 100 Brazilian cases, Feldmeier et al. found 68 female upper genital, and 32 lower genital localizations [16]. In Tanzania, 41.6% of 423 biopsy-diagnosed schistosomiasis were cases of female genital schistosomiasis [39]. Our study confirms the high female to male ratio of the infection, and the high rate of UGS in particular. We did not find an increased association of schistosomiasis and cervical pre-invasive or invasive lesions in HIV-infected women [30]. This may be due to the fact that the majority of our cases were infected with *S. hematobium*.

In Africa, two-thirds of infections are due to *S. haematobium*, the "neglected" schistosome [37-38]. The discrepancy between the magnitude of the endemicity of and the basic scientific knowledge about *S. haematobium* is due to the absence or shortage of animal models, the difficulty to maintain its life cycle in the laboratory, and *in vitro* systems [37-38]. However, the recent determination of its whole-genome sequence is a major progress in the understanding of the pathology and contribution to a potential vaccine [39]. The knowledge of the immunobiological interactions between HIV and schistosomes is also limited to *S. mansoni* [40]. Therefore, for the time being, preventive measures remain the mainstay to protect women from schistosome-related morbidity and mortality.

References

[1] Mbambazi, P.S., Andan, O., Fitzgerald, D.W., Chitsulo, L., Engels, D., Downs, J.A. (2011). Examining the relationship between urogenital schistosomiasis and HIV infection. *PLoS Negl Trop Dis* 5, e1396 doi:10.1371/journal.pntd.0001396.

[2] World Health Organization (2013). Schistosomiasis: number of people treated in 2011. *Weekly Epidemiological Record* 8, 81-88.

[3] Hotez, P. (2009) Empowering women and improving female reproductive health through control of neglected tropical diseases. *PLoS Negl Trop Dis* 3, e559.

[4] Hotez, P.J., Kamath, A. (2009). Neglected tropical diseases in sub-Saharan Africa: review of their prevalence, distribution, and disease burden. *Plos Negl Trop Dis* 3, e412.

[5] Information Resource Centre, World Health Organization (2010). Report of an informal working group meeting on urogenital schistosomiasis and HIV transmission, 1-2 October 2009. WHO, Geneva.

[6] Thomassen Morgas, D.E., Kvalsig, J.D., Gundersen, S.G., Taylor, M, Kjetland, E.F. (2010). Schistosomiasis and water-related practices in school girls in rural Kwazulu-Natal, South Africa. *South Afr J Epidemiol Infect* 25, 30-33.

[7] Meents, E.F., Boyles, T.H. (2010). Schistosoma haematobium prevalence in school children in the rural Eastern Cape Province, South Africa. *South Afr J Epidemiol Infect* 25, 28-29.

[8] World Health Organization (2009). Neglected Tropical Diseases. Statement – WHO working group on urogenital schistosomiasis and HIV transmission, 1-2 October 2009. Available at: http://www.who.int /neglected_diseases

[9] Stoever, K., Molyneux, D., Hotez, P., Fenwick, A. (2009). HIV/AIDS, schistosomiasis, and girls. *The Lancet* 373, 2025-2026.

[10] Berge, S.T., Kabatereine, N., Gundersen, S.G., Taylor, M., Kvalsig, J.D., Mkhize-Kwitshana, Z. et al. (2011). Generic praziquantel in South

Africa: the necessity for policy change to provide cheap, safe and efficacious schistosomiasis drugs for the poor, rural population. *South Afr J Epidemiol Infect* 26, 22-25.

[11] Höppli, R. (1932) Histological observations in experimental schistosomiasis. *Chin Med J* 46, 1179.

[12] Helling-Giese, G., Sjaastadt, A., Poggensee, G., Kjetland, E.F., Richter, J., Chitsulo, L. et al. (1996). Female genital schistosomiasis (FGS): relationship between gynecological and histopathological findings. *Acta Trop* 62, 257-267.

[13] Feldmeier, H., Correia Daccal, R., Martins, M.J., Soares, V., Martins, R. (1998). Genital manifestations of schistosoma mansoni in women: important but neglected. *Mem Inst Oswaldo Cruz* 1, 127-133.

[14] Kjetland, E.F., Ndhlovu, P.D., Mduluza, T., Gomo, E., Gwanzura, L., Mason, P.R., et al. (2005). Simple clinical manifestations of genital schistosoma haematobium infection in rural Zimbabwean women. *Am J Trop Med Hyg* 72, 311-319.

[15] Kjetland, E.F., Ten Hove, R.J., Gomo, E., Midzi, N., Gwanzura, L., Mason, P. et al., (2009). Schistosomiasis PCR in vaginal lavage as an indicator of genital schistosoma haematobium infection in rural Zimbabwean women. *Am J Trop Med Hyg* 81, 1050-1055.

[16] http://www.stats.sa.gov.za demography/vital statistics 2011.

[17] World Health Organization (2011) Schistosomiasis. Countries x indicators. Available at: http://www.who.int/neglected_diseases /preventive_chemotherapy/sch/db/index.html

[18] Mahmood, A.A.F., Adeh, A.F. (2000). Trematodes and other flukes. In: Mandell, Douglas, and Bennett's Principles and Practice of Infectious Diseases, 5th ed. New York, Churchill Livinstone 2950.

[19] McCully, R.M., Barron, C.N., Cheever, A.W. (1876). Schistosomiasis. In: Binford, C.H., Connor, C.H. (eds) Pathology of Tropical and Extraordinary Diseases. Washington, D.C.: Armed Forces Institute of Pathology, 482-508.

[20] Cooper, K., Haffajee, Z., Taylor, L. (1997). Human papillomavirus and schistosomiasis associated bladder cancer. *J Clin Pathol: Mol Pathol* 50, 145-148.

[21] Mostafa, M.H., Sheweita, S.A.,O'Connor, P.J. (1999). Relationship between schistosomiasis and bladder cancer. *Clin Microbiol Rev* 12, 97-111.

[22] Palumbo, E. Association between schistosomiasis and cancer: a review (2007). *Infect Dis Clin Pract* 15, 145-148.

[23] Bagwandeen, S.B. (1972). Carcinoma of the male breast in Zambia. *East Afr Med* J 48-49.
[24] van Bogaert, L.J. (2000). Male breast cancer in the Transkei region, South Africa. *Southern Afr J Epidemiol Infect* 15, 46-47.
[25] Szela, E., Bachicha, J., Miller, D., Till, M., Wilson, J.B. (1993). *Int J Gynecol Obstet* 42, 127-130.
[26] Moubayed, P., Ziehe, A., Peters, J., Mwakyoma, H., Schmidt, D. (1995). Carcinoma of the uterine cervix associated with schistosomiasis and human papillomaviruses. *Int J Gynecol Obstet* 49, 175-179.
[27] Petry, K.U., Scholz, U., Hollwitz, B., Von Wasielewski, R., Meijer, C. (2003). Human papillomavirus, coinfection with schistosoma haematobium, and cervical neoplasia in rural Tanzania. *Int J Gynecol Cancer* 13, 505-509.
[28] Richens, J. (2004). Genital manifestations of tropical diseases. *Sex Transm Infect* 80, 12-17.
[29] Poggensee, G., Kiwelu, I., Weger, V., Göppner, D., Diedrich, T., Krantz, I., Feldmeier, H. (2000). Female genital schistosomiasis of the lower genital tract: prevalence and disease-associated morbidity in Northern Tanzania. *J Infect Dis* 181, 1210-1213.
[30] Monsunjac, M.B., Tadros, T., Beach, R., Majumdar, B. (2003). Cervical schistosomiasis, human papilloma virus (HPV), and human immunodeficiency virus (HIV): a dangerous coexistence or coincidence? *Gynecol Oncol* 90, 211-214.
[31] Kjetland, E.F., Ndhlovu, P.D., Gomo, E., Mduluza, T, Midzi, N., Gwanzura, L. et al. (2006). Association between genital schistosomiasis and HIV in rural Zimbabwean women. *AIDS* 20, 593-600.
[32] Noblick, J., Skolnik, R., Hotez, P.J. (2011). Linking global HIV/AIDS treatments with national programs for the control and elimination of neglected tropical diseases. *PloS Negl Trop Dis* 5, e1022.
[33] Kallestrup, P., Zinyama, R., Gomo, E., Butterworth, A.E., Mudenge, B. et al. (2005). Schistosomiasis and HIV-1 infection in rural Zimbabwe: effect of treatment on CD4 count and plasma HIV-1 RNA load. *J Infect Dis* 192, 1956-1961.
[34] Badawy, A.H. (1962). Schistosomiasis of the cervix. *Br Med J* 1, 3-4.
[35] Swai, B., Poggensee, G., Mtweve, S., Krantz, A. (2006). Female genital schistosomiasis as an evidence of a neglected cause for reproductive ill-health: a retrospective histopathological study from Tanzania. *BMC Infect Dis* 6, 134.

[36] van Bogaert LJ (2013). Cervical neoplasia-associated schistosomiasis in HIV-infected and uninfected South African women. *J Genit Syst Dis* 2, 1.

[37] Brindley P, Hotez PJ (2013). Urogenital schistosomiasis and Schistosoma haematobium infection in the postgeneomic-era. *PLoS Negl Trop Dis* 7 (3): e1961.

[38] Rinaldi G, Okatcha TI, Propatiloff A, Ayuk MA, Suttiprapa S, Mann VH, et al. (2011). Genetic manipulation of schistosoma haematobium, the neglected schistosome. *PLoS Negl Trop Dis* 5 (10): e1348.

[39] Young ND, Jex AR, Li B, Liu S, Yang L, Xiong Z, et al. (2012). Whole-genome sequence of schistosoma haematobium. *Nature Genetics* 44 (2): 221-25.

[40] Mazigo HD, Nuwaha F, Wilson S, Kinung'hi S, Morona D, Waihenya R, et al. (2013). Epidemiology and interactions of human immunodeficiency virus-1 and Schistosoma mansoni in sub-Saharan Africa. *Inf Dis Poverty* 2(1): 2.

In: Schistosomiasis
Editor: Adriana Erica Miele
ISBN: 978-1-63117-186-4

Chapter 8

Epidemiology of Imported Bilharzia: Prophylactic and Treatment Options for Children

José Uberos Fernández*[1*]*, Antonio Molina-Carballo*[1]*,
Manuel Molina-Oya*[2]*, Eduardo Narbona-López*[1]
and Antonio Muñoz-Hoyos*[1]
[1]Paediatrics Service, San Cecilio University Hospital, Granada, Spain
[2]Granada Metropolitan Sanitary District, Granada, Spain

Abstract

In its resolution WHA54.19 (2001), the WHO urged Member States "...to ensure access to essential drugs against schistosomiasis...in all health services in endemic areas for the treatment of clinical cases and groups at high risk of morbidity such as women and children, with the goal of attaining a minimum target of regular administration of chemotherapy to at least 75% and up to 100% of all school-age children at risk of morbidity by 2010". However, the number of countries considered endemic for schistosomiasis increased from 77 in 2010 to 78 in 2011 and treatment was only guaranteed in 52 of these countries.

* Corresponding Author address: Dr. José Uberos. c/Málaga 1, 18170 Alfacar, Granada (Spain). Fax: +34 958 240740. email: juberos@ugr.es.

According to WHO data, in 2012 over 111 million school-age children were in need of preventive chemotherapy.

It is estimated that urinary schistosomiasis (bilharzia) annually affects 200 million people, of whom 120 million remain asymptomatic and at least 200,000 die from related causes. In Spain and in many other European countries, immigrants from areas endemic for S. haematobium regularize their employment status by periodically visiting their countries of origin. This circumstance requires a thorough anamnesis to be conducted, inquiring in each case into the trips made in recent months. This information continues to be the most important element required for a presumptive diagnosis and the factor motivating the search for S. haematobium eggs in a urine sample to confirm the diagnosis.

In January 2008, Spain had 5.2 million registered foreign residents, 11.3% of the total population, as well as a large population that does not appear in any record, but is estimated at over 400,000 people. More than half of these people come from low-income countries and endemic areas for schistosomiasis. These numbers have declined in the last year, partly due to the economic crisis affecting the European Union.

The epidemiology of urinary schistosomiasis and the incidence of infection vary considerably among geographic areas. They are believed to be related to the population density of freshwater snails, especially the species Biomphalaria and Bulinus, the density of cercariae in contaminated water and the frequency of human contact with such water. The snail species involved in the transmission may have prolonged survival at mean temperatures above 18°C, a circumstance that is considered particularly important in the transmission of the disease.

To date, few published studies on imported schistosomiasis have had an adequate sample size and, in any case, differ in their definition of the diagnosis, clinical presentation and source of infection. In most published series, diagnosis is performed by antibody titer, because the parasite load is usually too low to enable identification in urine. In fact, most chronically infected patients may remain asymptomatic. The epidemiological and clinical impact of schistosomiasis in immigrants from endemic regions differs considerably from that seen in Western visitors to endemic areas. While most infected immigrants remain asymptomatic, with a low parasite load, the exposed Western population more frequently develops Katayama syndrome with more evident clinical signs and symptoms.

This chapter reviews the epidemiology of schistosomiasis in Western countries, the mechanisms involved in its transmission and the prophylactic and treatment options for children affected by it.

Keywords: Imported schistosomiasis, epidemiology in non-endemic areas, diagnosis in children

Introduction

Schistosomiasis is a parasitic disease caused by a trematode helminth of the genus *Schistosoma*. Only six species affect humans: *S. haematobium, S. mansoni, S. japonicum, S. intercalatum, S. mekongi* and *S. malayensis*. It is also termed bilharziasis, after its discoverer, the German doctor Theodor Maximillian Bilharz. In 1851, during his work at the Egyptian Department of Hygiene, he discovered this new class of helminth in the vena cava blood of patients who had died of haematuria.

Bilharzia is a major public health problem that affects approximately 200 million people each year, of whom at least 80% live in Africa [16]. In many Western countries, immigrants from areas endemic for *S. haematobium* regularize their employment status by periodically visiting their home countries, where reinfection may occur. This circumstance requires a thorough anamnesis to be conducted, inquiring in each case into the trips made in recent months. This information continues to be the most important element required for a presumptive diagnosis and is the factor motivating the search for *S. hematobium* eggs in a urine sample to confirm the diagnosis or as part of a serological investigation in cases of long-term haematuria.

The Biological Cycle of the Genus Schistosoma

Schistosoma has a cylindrical body, ending in two oral suckers (See also Chapter 1). There are two main forms of schistosomiasis: intestinal and urogenital. Among the species that parasitise humans, only *S. haematobium* affects the urogenital apparatus, with the other species normally producing intestinal parasitisation (Figure 1). The adult forms are hematophagous, and, in the definitive host, are found in the venous plexuses, especially the mesenteric (*S. mansoni, S. japonicum, S. intercalatum, S. mekongi*) or perivesical ones (*S.haematobium*). The couple migrates here through the capillaries and venules, where the female ponds 100-1000 eggs a day. These eggs, in turn, migrate through the walls of the vessels in which they were deposited, reaching the tissues and then either the intestinal lumen or the urinary bladder lumen. Finally, they emerge in the faeces or the urine, respectively.

Transported in the faeces or urine, the embryo eggs contaminate waters in rivers, lakes and irrigated fields, where in a few hours they hatch and release the miracidia.

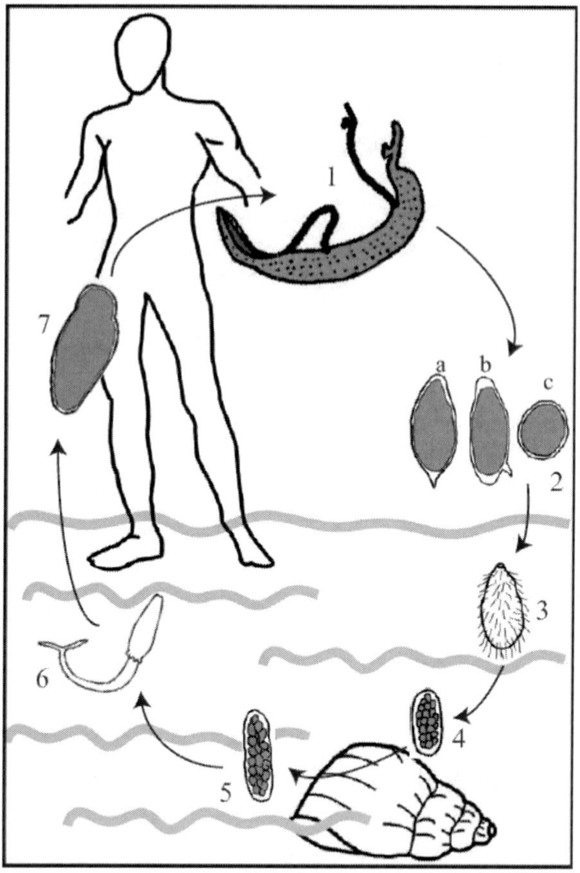

Figure 1. The life cycle of schistosomes, with a morphological description of the different life stages. Adult worms pair (1) living in the definitive human host blood (periportal veins for those species causing intestinal schistosomiasis; peri-bladder veins for those causing urogenital schistosomiasis). Each female lays 20-1000 eggs/day, depending on the species. The eggs (2) are recognizable by their morphology: (a) *S. haematobium* eggs present a terminal spine, (b) *S. mansoni* eggs have a lateral spine; (c) *S. japonicum* eggs are round. The eggs are excreted by either faeces (b,c) or urine (a). Once they reach a freshwater source, they hatch into a free-living ciliated stage called miracidium (3). This one swims towards the mollusc host and penetrates it. Inside the freshwater snails asexual reproduction takes place to increase the number of parasites. Two sequential life stages arise from the miracidium: the mother (4) and the daughter sporocyst (5). This last releases into the water thousands of caudated free living cercariae (6), which are the infective stage for the human host. Cercariae are able to penetrate intact human skin and to develop into a juvenile form: the schistosomulum (7), which migrates undisturbed from the derma to the lungs, where it sexually matures into the adult form (1). This last migrates to the final destination, where it can live for up to 30 years.

The latter penetrate and parasitise certain snails that inhabit the fresh water and constitute the intermediary host. Each species of *Schistosoma* parasitises a particular genus of snail, as follows:

- *S. haematobium*:. Bulinus spp, Physopis spp, Planorbis spp.
- *S. mansoni*: Biomphalaria.
- *S. japonicum*: Oncomelania.
- *S. mekongi*: Tricula aperta.
- *S. intercalatum*: Bulinus.
- *S. malayensis*: Tricula aperta.

Within the snail, the miracidia mature for approximately 6 weeks to become cercariae (with a bifurcated tail and penetration glands), which are then released back into the water. Humans can become infected by walking, bathing or washing in water contaminated by cercariae, which adhere to the skin and penetrate it. In this process, they lose their tails and are transformed into schistosomulae, which reach the bloodstream and are systemically distributed, reaching the lungs and finally the liver, where they mature into the adult form and attach themselves in their definitive location, the mesenteric or vesical venous plexuses, and thus the cycle is completed. The period between the cercariae penetrating the skin and the beginning of egg production from adult worms is 4-7 weeks. Adult worms can live in the venous plexuses for 20-30 years. Direct transmission between persons does not take place, as the participation of the snail in the biological cycle of this trematode is absolutely mandatory [20].

Epidemiological Questions

According to WHO data [22], with the independence of South Sudan in 2011, the number of schistosomiasis-endemic countries has increased from 77 in 2010 to 78 in 2011. Large-scale treatment is only ensured in 52 of these countries. The rate of transmission of schistosomiasis is considered low in 7 countries and needs to be verified in 19. The figures published by the WHO in its 2012 report [22] indicate that at least 243 million persons required preventive chemoprophylaxis in 2011. Large-scale schistosomiasis control measures continue to require further resources for treatment programmes, water purification, the provision of health resources and health education and measures to control aquatic snails.

In some countries, the interruption of schistosomiasis transmission can only be achieved through improved hygienic-sanitary conditions and actions to control the aquatic snail population [5]. The WHO, in its WHA65.21 report, acknowledged the progress made in controlling the disease and highlighted the need to verify the results of ongoing programmes to interrupt the transmission of the disease. In 2011, 28 million people received treatment for schistosomiasis, of whom 58% were children aged 5-14 years. Unfortunately, data are only available for treatments performed in 46% of the schistosomiasis-endemic countries. Available data indicate that in 2011, the number of persons treated was 20% lower than in 2010, possibly not due to a lower incidence of the disease, but rather to the fact that 8 countries that reported data in 2010 did not do so in 2011 (Figure 2).

Children, who may play in infected water, and who often suffer a hygiene deficit, are particularly vulnerable. Also at risk are women who carry out domestic tasks, such as washing clothes in these waters. It has been estimated that in chronic cases of vaginal schistosomiasis, the risk of HIV infection is multiplied by three-fold [12].

The WHO strategies for controlling schistosomiasis are centred on reducing cases of the disease *via* periodic, focused treatment with praziquantel. This is a cheap and effective drug, costing only €0.08 per dose. Nevertheless, it may still be expensive for the health administrations of some developing countries. Outbreaks of schistosomiasis can be identified by haematuria screening of schoolchildren and, in cases of epidemic, treating the entire community at risk [4].

The epidemiology of urinary schistosomiasis and the incidence of infection vary widely among geographical areas, but they are considered to be related to the population density of freshwater snails, especially the species *Biomphalaria* and *Bulinus.*

Other relevant factors are the density of cercariae in the contaminated water and the frequency of human contact with such water. The snail species involved in the transmission may have prolonged survival at average temperatures above 18°C, and this circumstance is considered particularly important in the disease transmission. Current opinion is that transmission by both snail species occurs not only in rivers and lakes, but also by means of irrigation systems, which can play an important role in local endemic schistosomiasis.

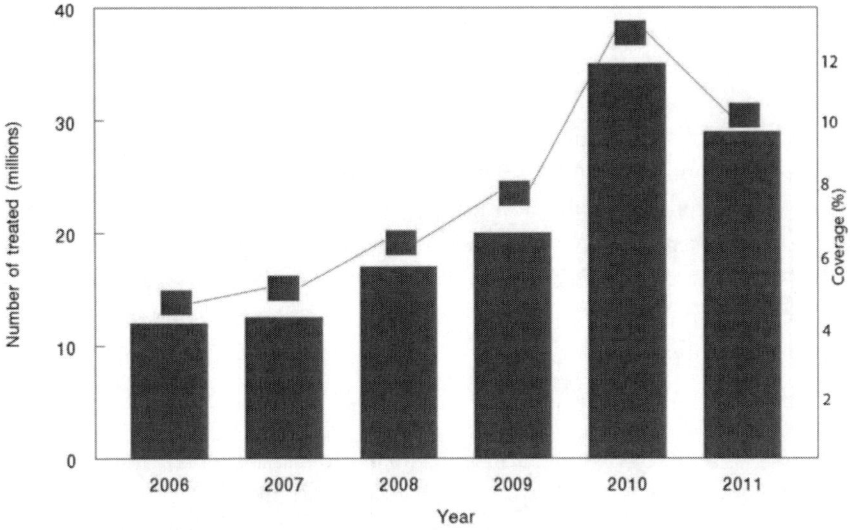

Figure 2. Number of people treated for schistosomiasis and reported coverage of treatment (%), data extracted from WHO Region, 2006–2011.

With respect to exposure to schistosomiasis, there are considerable differences between the local population and foreign workers or immigrants on a holiday visit to their countries of origin. Among the latter, exposure tends to be occasional, short-term and related to recreational water activities.

The GeoSentinel Surveillance Network carried out a transversal study of affected travellers who had visited endemic schistosomiasis areas between 1997 and 2008. The GeoSentinel is a worldwide communication and data collection network for the surveillance of travel related morbidity. Confirmed cases were communicated in 12 countries belonging to this worldwide surveillance network. In a total sample of 25,240 people, some 410 persons (16‰) were found to be suffering from schistosomiasis; 37% were European, 24% North American, 24% Asian and 15% from Oceania. Over 80% of those affected had acquired this disease in Africa, mainly in sub-Saharan Africa. There were some differences depending on demographic characteristics and the type of travel. Male travellers and travellers aged under 45 years were more likely to be diagnosed with schistosomiasis than with another illness. When the data were controlled for age and sex, those traveling for missionary or other volunteer work were twice as likely to be diagnosed with schistosomiasis than were tourists and other types of travellers. Business travellers were less likely to be diagnosed with schistosomiasis than were tourists and other types of travellers. Individuals traveling as expatriates, regardless of the type of travel, were twice as likely to be diagnosed with schistosomiasis as those staying for shorter times and staying in hotels. Attending a pre-travel health care consultation was also associated with being diagnosed with schistosomiasis. 63% of the 401 travellers, who were infected with schistosomiasis, on their return attended a GeoSentinel clinic within six months of return, with a median time-to-presentation of six weeks (interquartile range IQR 2–12 weeks); the median duration of travel for this group was 13 weeks (IQR 4–33 weeks). 110 (27%) travellers attended a GeoSentinel clinic more than 6 months after their return. Time to presentation was 6-24 months for 73 travellers (18%), 3-4 years for 16 (4%), and five or more years for 18 (4%). 41% of the 319 travellers who were asymptomatic at presentation were diagnosed with schistosomiasis. The most commonly reported symptoms were gastrointestinal, fever, urogenital and fatigue. Returned travellers with schistosomiasis were more likely to present with fever than those who were ruled out for schistosomiasis. Those with *S. haematobium* and *S. mansoni* infections presented with more respiratory symptoms than did those ruled out for schistosomiasis. Moreover, returned travellers with schistosomiasis who were seen within six months of travel more often presented with fever and respiratory symptoms compared with those who presented later [13].

Imported travel-related infections were also studied in a retrospective and descriptive study of travellers returning from the tropics and attended at the Tropical Medicine Unit, Infectious Diseases Department of Hospital Ramon y Cajal in Madrid (Spain) during the period January 1989 to November 2006. A total of 2982 travellers were analysed; 1387 had travelled to Sub-Saharan Africa and 44 of these were diagnosed with schistosomiasis (3%). 98% of the patients with schistosomiasis had travelled to Sub-Saharan Africa and only 2% to other geographical areas [20].

Many centres in Australia routinely screen African refugees for schistosomiasis using serology, and in some cases with faeces and urine examination for schistosome eggs. A seroprevalence of 38% was reported for 653 African refugee adults and children arriving in Australia, predominantly from Liberia, Burundi, Tanzania and Sudan. A multivariate analysis of the Newcastle data showed that schistosomiasis serology was much more likely to be positive among those from East Africa (OR 14.5) and West Africa (OR 5.5) than those from the Sudan region (OR 1.0) [10].

In most published series, diagnosis is performed by antibody titer, because the parasite load is usually too low to enable identification in urine. In fact, most chronically infected patients may remain asymptomatic. The epidemiological and clinical impact of schistosomiasis in immigrants from endemic regions differs considerably from that seen in Western visitors to endemic areas. While most infected immigrants remain asymptomatic, with a low parasite load, the exposed Western population more frequently develops Katayama syndrome with more evident clinical signs and symptoms.

Important Aspects for Diagnosis

According to all health care protocols for immigrant children, the presence of *S. haematobium* should be considered in cases of persistent haematuria. This is also applicable to children born in Western countries from immigrant families, who periodically visit their home countries. We have observed such a case, of a child with Spanish nationality, born from immigrant parents [19]. There are increasing references to urinary schistosomiasis diagnosed among immigrants living in Western countries [6, 11].

The disease is acquired by contact with fresh water contaminated with *S. haematobium* cercariae. In non-sensitized subjects, the penetration of cercariae through the skin may cause transient pruritic dermatitis. 3-4 weeks later, there is a febrile reaction with headache, joint pain, swollen liver and spleen, diarrhoea and eosinophilia, known as the Katayama syndrome. In 37% of patients with acute schistosomiasis, symptoms appear 3 weeks after exposure (3.1 ± 2.7 weeks). Fever is the most prevalent symptom, followed by respiratory symptoms and rash. Only 9.5% of cases present the full range of symptoms of acute schistosomiasis. 20% of patients have chronic schistosomiasis at the time of diagnosis, and the lag time from exposure to diagnosis ranges from 4 months to 3 years. Moreover, 47% of infected patients remain asymptomatic [8].

The immune response to early-stage schistosomiasis may be Th1-type, developing to Th2 after egg laying by mature worms [2]. The Th2 response is controlled by the IgE response, which stimulates the eosinophils to release cytokines against the schistosome. During infection, as well as the IgE response, IgG4 infection occurs, which potentially blocks the effect of other immunoglobulins. In the host, the most intense inflammatory response does not take place against the schistosome antigens, but rather against the eggs trapped in the tissues, which provoke the formation of mucosal granulomatous hyperplasias, together with nodules and polyps that tend to ulcerate and bleed

[7, see also chapter 2]. T cell-mediated immunity is crucial to the development of resistance to schistosome re-infection.

Initially, parasitisation may be asymptomatic, followed by haematuria which is more intense at the end of urination and may be accompanied by dysuria. The existence of haematuria at the end of urination is related to the presence of viable eggs deposited on the bladder wall, related to lengthy processes with the presence of granulomas in the bladder submucosa and distal ureter [18]. Advanced stages of the disease may give rise to hydronephrosis caused by ureteral obstruction and peri-vesical calcifications. In repeated and severe infections, the ureteral wall mucosa is also affected, and obstructive uropathy and hydronephrosis may evolve.

Eosinophilia is a nonspecific finding observed in 57% of cases. In patients with symptoms of acute schistosomiasis or Katayama syndrome, the prevalence of eosinophilia may be slightly higher, up to 61% in some series [3]. The correlation of eosinophilia with positive serological data can be relatively low (19%), while with negative serological data it is somewhat higher (43%). In patients with chronic schistosomiasis, eosinophilia is uncommon. Direct microscopic examination of urine reveals schistosome eggs in only 22% of patients with urinary schistosomiasis, and in Western countries this has a low correlation (13%) with positive serological data [3].

In our society, schistosomiasis screening for people at risk should be done as a serological test, conducted at least 6 weeks after potential exposure to contaminated water. In this period, the absence of antibodies against schistosomes virtually excludes the possibility of infection. When schistosome serology is positive, the identification of eggs in urine is indicated, although the low sensitivity of this test needs to be taken into account [21].

Treatment and Prophylaxis

For over 20 years, the most effective means of controlling the disease has been chemoprophylaxis with praziquantel. In endemic areas, the WHO recommends collective treatment of the population with praziquantel (Table 1 lists the recommended treatment strategies [5]). In addition, many African countries such as Ghana have concentrated efforts to combat schistosomiasis by controlling the vectors (snails) in the rivers.

The treatment of choice is praziquantel at a dose of 40 mg/Kg per day in two doses, every 12 hours. With this dose, the 6-week cure rate is 88%; the administration of a second dose of praziquantel at 4-6 weeks increases the cure rate to 100% [9]. During the immature stages, schistosomes are moderately refractory to praziquantel, but their sensitivity to treatment increases with maturity and egg laying. In consequence, during the first 10-12 weeks after *S. haematobium* infection, praziquantel may not be useful [17].

In endemic areas, reinfection after praziquantel treatment is common. Today, it is recognized that reinfection with *S. haematobium* is closely related to the IgE/IgG4 balance [7]. Although at present there is no evidence of the existence of strains resistant to praziquantel, a reduction in susceptibility to the drug has been reported [17]. Praziquantel combines safety and low price, and is active against the adult stages of schistosomes. One of the major limitations of praziquantel is its non-efficacy against immature stages, which is related to treatment failure and a higher frequency of reinfection. Large-scale schistosomiasis control programmes depend on the use of praziquantel, and there is concern that its continued use could lead to the development of resistance in the parasite.

Table 1. WHO recommended treatment strategy for schistosomiasis in preventive chemotherapy

Prevalence* in school-age children (SAC)	Treatment Group	Target Group	Treatment Frequency
≥50%	A (High)	Treat all SAC and adults at risk	Once every year
≥10% and <50%	B (Medium)	Treat all SAC and adults at risk	Once every 2 years
≥1% and <10%	C (Low)	Treat all SAC	Once every 3 years (twice during primary schooling age)

**Determined by parasitological methods*

The schistosomicide activity of artemisinin was discovered in the 1980s. Its activity is directed against the immature stages of the parasite, and so this would complement the therapeutic activity of praziquantel. This has led some authors to propose the combined use of praziquantel and artemisinin as a treatment strategy for schistosomiasis. In this respect, Pérez del Villar and co-workers [14] conducted a systematic review, analysing the available data on the safety and efficacy of artemisinin in the treatment and prophylaxis of schistosomiasis, examining 50 articles of the 261 published on the question. Seven studies compared artemisinin with praziquantel and reported a lower cure rate for artemisinin. Four studies evaluated the combination of artemisinin and praziquantel *versus* praziquantel alone. In urinary schistosomiasis, the patients treated with the combination presented higher cure rates than those treated with praziquantel alone (OR=1.84, 95% confidence interval (CI) 1.01-3.36, p=0.047). These observations are also applicable to *S. mansoni* and *S. japonicum*. Three studies compared artemisinin and sulfadoxine-pyrimethamine with praziquantel alone, and found that the cure rate for the combination therapy was significantly lower than that for praziquantel alone. Finally, five studies compared artemisinin with a placebo treatment and observed a better response with the artemisinin (OR=0.11, 95% CI 0.06 - 0.22, p=0.001).

The side effects most frequently described after the use of artemisinin are epigastric pain, headache, nausea and vomiting. Nevertheless, all studies agree that both praziquantel and artemisinin are in general well tolerated.

At present, it is concluded that artemisinin used as the sole treatment option is not recommended, as it is mainly effective against the immature forms of the parasite, and its cure rates are lower than those of praziquantel. Furthermore, its use in combination with praziquantel raises the question of whether more widespread use could facilitate the emergence of resistance in the treatment of malaria.

The above considerations regarding treatment reflect the need to achieve approaches that are more specific and which provide long-term protection against schistosomiasis. The development of a vaccine strategy seems appropriate though it would need longer times to be achieved. Although several vaccine candidates have been proposed, the antigen glutathione S-transferase 28 kDa (Sh28GST) has been well characterized, and the immunization of diverse laboratory animals with this antigen has produced a significant decrease in the fertility of the parasite, and the safety of the procedure has been demonstrated [1]. Some studies have shown that resistance to reinfection is associated with the presence of antibodies to 28GST, capable of inhibiting the 28GST enzymatic activity of the parasite. Riveau and co-workers [15] published a phase I clinical trial focusing on the safety and tolerability of recombinant Sh28GST vaccine, adjuvated with aluminium hydroxide (rSh28GST) in humans. For ethical reasons, the authors recruited an adult population, although it seems clear that children would constitute the ideal population for this vaccine. These authors concluded that the recombinant vaccine (rSh28GST) adjuvated with aluminium hydroxide was both safe and tolerable for adults.

Conclusion

There are increasing references to urinary schistosomiasis diagnosed among immigrants living in Western countries. The schistosomiasis screening for people at risk should be done as a serological test, conducted at least 6 weeks after a potential exposure to contaminated waters. In this period, the absence of antibodies against schistosomes virtually excludes the possibility of infection. Should the schistosome serology be positive, the identification of eggs in urine would be indicated, although the low sensitivity of this test needs to be taken into account. The treatment of choice is praziquantel. Although at present there is no evidence of the existence of strains resistant to praziquantel. In endemic areas, reinfection after praziquantel treatment is very common. Therefore in school children the frequency of prophylactic treatment with praziquantel should be adjusted to the prevalence of the disease in their environment.

References

[1] Balloul JM, Sondermeyer P, Dreyer D, Capron M, Grzych JM, Pierce RJ, Carvallo D, Lecocq JP, Capron A. 1987. Molecular cloning of a protective antigen of schistosomes. *Nature* 326: 149-153.

[2] Bergquist R 2008. A century of schistosomiasis research. *Acta Trop* 108: 65-68.

[3] Bierman WF, Wetsteyn JC, van GT 2005. Presentation and diagnosis of imported schistosomiasis: relevance of eosinophilia, microscopy for ova, and serology. *J Travel Med* 12: 9-13.

[4] Hotez PJ, Engels D, Fenwick A, Savioli L. 2010. Africa is desperate for praziquantel. *Lancet* 376: 496-498.

[5] Kabore A, Biritwum NK, Downs PW, Soares Magalhaes RJ, Zhang Y, Ottesen EA. 2013. Predictive vs. empiric assessment of schistosomiasis: implications for treatment projections in Ghana. *PLoS Negl Trop Dis* 7: e2051.

[6] Maese Heredia, R, Rubi Palomares, I, Peña Muñoz, M, Bueno Fernández, A, Weil Lara, B. 2009. Hematuria recurrente. *An Pediatr (Barc.)* 57: 501-502.

[7] McManus DP, Loukas A. 2008. Current status of vaccines for schistosomiasis. *Clin. Microbiol. Rev.* 21: 225-242.

[8] Meltzer E, Artom G, Marva E, Assous MV, Rahav G, Schwartz E. 2006. Schistosomiasis among travelers: New aspects of an old disease. *Emerg. Infect Dis.* 12: 1696-1700.

[9] Midzi N, Sangweme D, Zinyowera S, Mapingure MP, Brouwer KC, Kumar N, Mutapi F, Woelk G, Mduluza T. 2008. Efficacy and side effects of praziquantel treatment against Schistosoma haematobium infection among primary school children in Zimbabwe. *Trans R Soc Trop Med Hyg* 102: 759-766.

[10] Murray R, Davis J, Biggs V-A, Krause V. 2009. Diagnosis, management and prevention of infections in recently arrived refugees. Dreamweaver Publishing Pty Ltd.,

[11] Navarro Cabañas, G., Garcia Sanchez, N., Rubio Rubio, R., Izaguirre Zugazaga, C., Clavel Parrilla, A., Seral García, C. 2006. Esquistosomiasis urogenital: un diagnóstico sencillo. *An Pediatr (Barc.)* 64: 290-291.

[12] Ndhlovu PD, Mduluza T, Kjetland EF, Midzi N, Nyanga L, Gundersen SG, Friis H, Gomo E. 2007. Prevalence of urinary schistosomiasis and HIV in females living in a rural community of Zimbabwe: does age matter? *Trans R Soc Trop Med Hyg* 101: 433-438.

[13] Nicolls DJ, Weld LH, Schwartz E, Reed C, von SF, Freedman DO, Kozarsky PE. 2008. Characteristics of schistosomiasis in travelers reported to the GeoSentinel Surveillance Network 1997-2008. *Am J Trop Med Hyg* 79: 729-734.

[14] Perez d, V, Burguillo FJ, Lopez-Aban J, Muro A. 2012. Systematic review and meta-analysis of artemisinin based therapies for the treatment and prevention of schistosomiasis. *PLoS ONE* 7: e45867.

[15] Riveau G, Deplanque D, Remoue F, Schacht AM, Vodougnon H, Capron M, Thiry M, Martial J, Libersa C, Capron A. 2012. Safety and Immunogenicity of rSh28GST Antigen in Humans: Phase 1 Randomized Clinical Study of a Vaccine Candidate against Urinary Schistosomiasis. *PLoS Negl Trop Dis* 6: e1704.

[16] Rotger M, Serra T, de Cardenas MG, Morey A, Vicente MA. 2004. Increasing incidence of imported schistosomiasis in Mallorca, Spain. *Eur. J. Clin. Microbiol Infect Dis* 23: 855-856.

[17] Sabra AN, Botros SS. 2008. Response of Schistosoma mansoni isolates having different drug sensitivity to praziquantel over several life cycle passages with and without therapeutic pressure. *J. Parasitol.* 94: 537-541.

[18] Tzanetou K, Adamis G, Andipa E, Zorzos C, Ntoumas K, Armenis K, Kontogeorgos G, Malamou-Lada E, Gargalianos P. 2007. Urinary tract Schistosoma haematobium infection: a case report. *J. Travel Med* 14: 334-337.

[19] Uberos J, Gamarra M, Prados E, Narbona-Lopez E. 2010. Importance of anamnesis in the diagnosis of urinary schistosomiasis. *An Pediatr (Barc)* 73: 214-216.

[20] Uberos J, Jerez-Calero A. 2012. Imported Schistosomiasis. In: Rokni MB (ed) Schistosomiasis. 171-182.

[21] Van GT, Vetter H, Vervoort T, Doenhoff MJ, Wetsteyn J, Overbosch D. 2002. Serodiagnosis of imported schistosomiasis by a combination of a commercial indirect hemagglutination test with *Schistosoma mansoni* adult worm antigens and an enzyme-linked immunosorbent assay with *S. mansoni* egg antigens. *J. Clin. Microbiol* 40: 3432-3437.

[22] W.H.O. 2013. *Schistosomiasis.* Weekly epidemiological record 88: 81-88.

Index

A

B

C

D

E

F

G

H

R

S

T

U

V

W

Z